The Alzheimer's Alternative

Researched Remedies that are Effective
in the Treatment
of Alzheimer's and other Dementias.

Steffan H. Abel D.C, M.Sc.

DISCLAIMER

No part of this publication may be reproduced or transmitted in any form or by any means, electronic or mechanical, including recording, photocopying, or via a computerised or electric storage or retrieval system without permission granted in writing from the author.

Although all the information contained herein is obtained from sources believed to be reliable its accuracy cannot be guaranteed. All material in this publication is provided for information only and may not be construed as medical advice or instruction. No action or inaction should be taken based solely on the contents of this publication; instead, readers should consult appropriate health professionals on any matter relating to their health and well being.

The information and opinions provided in this publication are believed to be accurate and sound, based on the best judgement available to the author, and readers who fail to consult with the appropriate health authorities assume the risk of any injuries. The author is not responsible for errors or omissions.

Dedication

to Dad

the reason behind this book.

to Mum

the reasoning behind this book.

to Sue

the reason for being here.

I would also like to acknowledge all the driving forces
that have been behind me throughout life
(although sometimes I wish they had been out in front!)
- too many to name but hopefully they all know who they are.

About The Author

Dr. Steffan H. Abel D.C. graduated from the Anglo-European College of Chiropractic in 1990 and since that time has had his own successful private practice in the North East of England.

Having parents that were both teachers and lecturers led him to developing both an open and enquiring mind. Since establishing his clinic he has had a tremendous and vested interest in trying to find and combine the best healing techniques so that he could offer the ultimate treatment to his patients.

To this end he has studied Hypnotherapy, N.L.P. and qualified as a Life Coach. He has also studied various Chiropractic-based treatments (gaining a M.Sc. in post graduate Clinical Chiropractic in 2003) as well as energy therapies such as Seichem and Reiki. In 2001 he became a Fellow of the College of Chiropractors and a Fellow of the Association of Osteomyology and in 2007 became a Fellow of the European Academy of Chiropractic.

He first encountered T.B.M. over 10 years ago and was so impressed with the technique that the urge to study it and if possible develop it further arose. This culminated in development of his own technique – Integrated Healing Systems – which he continues work on to this day.

In his spare time he spends between 15 and 25 hours per week researching all areas of "alternative" and allopathic healthcare in order to bring the best advice to his patients through his practice and writing and when not working he is to be found enjoying life with his partner – whom he loves tremendously!

Introduction

There are really only two things that will drive a researcher on and spur them to find out as much as they can about a particular subject. These are:

1. When there is the threat of a global epidemic that will affect millions of people, or
2. When a relative or a loved one is affected by a certain condition.

This book was hastened to its completion and publication for both of these reasons.

Initially it started out as a purely personal mission to make improvements in my own family. My father was diagnosed with Alzheimer's eight years ago and realising the progressive nature of the disease I looked at all the treatments available (both medically and complementary) which would be of help to him.

Also the expected numbers of sufferers from Alzheimer's disease is expected to quadruple in the very near future. Although no-one is sure why or what to do about it, everyone is clear about the suffering and the burden that this increase will have not only on those that develop the condition but their families, loved ones and those that look after and care for them.

I have spent many years looking at the various treatments and supplements that are available for the treatment of Alzheimer's and this is a distillation of the material that I have uncovered. These are the techniques that I have found to be most beneficial not only for my own circumstances but also that have helped my patients the most with their own families.

The research into Alzheimer's disease is ongoing and new ideas, treatments and theories are constantly coming to the attention of doctor's, support organisations and the media. Therefore, this book will constantly grow. All the latest advances will be collected and reviewed and if they are deemed to be of merit they will be uploaded to the website (to which you have free access with the purchase of this book) and will be added to further published editions with each new printing.

If you have any thoughts or contributions that you would like to see included please drop me an email. If suitable they will be entered on to the site and shared with others.

A quick glance though this book will show you that it is divided into eight sections. The first section is a brief overview of Alzheimer's disease – the history behind the condition, its probable causes, its effects, standard medical treatments and so forth. It is a short section that gives you a little background into the condition and whilst not compulsory (you won't lose any of the benefits you may gain from this book by skipping this section), I feel it is always useful to have a little information about what you are dealing with so that you are fully prepared. I believe that knowledge is power and the more you know about a subject the better you can deal with it.

The second and third sections will show how the effects of lifestyle can impact on the development of Alzheimer's disease and dementia – and more importantly show you simple steps you can take to prevent it.

Sections four and five will cover the nutritional aspects of preventing and improving dementia and Alzheimer's disease. These will cover vitamin supplements, herbal supplements and other supplements that have been shown to be of benefit.

These four sections combined will explain in detail how lifestyle changes, change of diet and how each of the nutritional supplements works. The individual studies that prove each treatment are described (and they are also referenced later).

Recommendation

Throughout the book you will find these little recommendation boxes. These are designed to give you a very brief summary of the dosages of the various supplements that have been suggested and action steps that you may like to take / implement.

Although this material is important (it is always best to know as much as you can about a condition before you tackle it) it is "harder going" and may not be that necessary to the reader who wants the solutions and wants them immediately to hand so that brings us to the sixth section of the book.

Here you will find a summary of all the nutritional advice, lifestyle changes and modifications that you can make that will have an effect on Alzheimer's. It is a summary that will inform you what is available, what are the best dosages or ways to implement the advice (should you so wish to do so) and if there are any possible side-effects or cautionary information you may need to be aware of.

Because there are varying opinions about what the actual cause of the condition is, the information will be collected into groups that tackle a specific area. These areas will be lifestyle, nutritional, hormonal, heavy metal poisoning and so on. If, for example, you believe that the problem is caused by one major factor look at the table for that factor and it will give you the related treatments that will improve it.

I personally believe that Alzheimer's is multi-factorial and it has many components to it – all of which will play a part to some degree or other. Therefore I prefer the shotgun approach and tend to use multiple treatments to tackle the condition. I am not that worried as to what brings about the improvement – as long as there is some!

The seventh section of the book is a compendium of useful contact organisations including both those that can give further advice on the subject and those that can offer support to the sufferer, their families and carers. The final section (section 8) includes all the references which are included to prove scientifically that there is help available.

The book that you are now holding contains all the information you will need on the latest treatments for warding off *and* slowing the progression of Alzheimer's disease. Compiled within these pages are practical tips on diet, lifestyle and supplements (including vitamins, minerals and herbs) all of which will improve you health and memory. All the supplements suggested are readily available from most health food shops or over the Internet.

Although, I have had very good results using the information you now have in your hands, every case is different. For this reason, I would urge you to seek advice from elsewhere (including your healthcare provider) before using any of the many good ideas you will find here especially if you are already taking prescribed medications. It is also important to remember that all supplements work differently with everyone, and it is impossible to say which ones may work best for you or even how long it may be before you notice any changes. Some may take a few days and some may take a few months to have an effect – but they will all help.

Because there is ongoing research into Alzheimer's disease and dementia no one book can ever be up to date. For this reason a website to accompany this book has been developed to include any new information as and when it occurs. Your purchase of this book allows you access to the members area of the www.alzheimersalternative.com website using the following log in information:

Log in name: information
Password: updates

A donation from the profits of the sale of this book will also be made to the Crossroads organisation which is a charity that provides help and support for carers and a running total of these donations can also be found on the website.

In closing I wish you every success implementing your new found knowledge and I hope that you are equally as pleased with the outcomes as I have been.

Dr. Steffan H. Abel D.C., M.Sc.

New to the 2nd Edition

- Further Brain Training Exercises.

- Information on the Importance of Phosphatidylserine.

- Information on wormwood supplementation.

- 3 more books you may wish to investigate for further information and ideas.

Section One

Alzheimer's in the U.K.

Before I move into the treatment aspect of the book I feel it would be beneficial to give you a little background on the condition. Although, this information is not vital to your treatment programme I feel it is important to fully understand the condition so that you can more easily grasp why it is so vitally important that you are aware of every step that can be taken to slow and prevent the disease.

Alzheimer's disease was named after Alois Alzheimer (1864–1915) who discovered plaques in the brain of a female that had died of dementia in the early 1900's. Although the condition was named after him following a presentation he gave in 1907, there were actually reported cases of similar conditions as early as 1887. Since then Alzheimer's has become recognised as one of the most common forms of dementia particularly in the elderly.

Alzheimer's disease affects around 420,000 people in the UK (and currently about 26 million people worldwide) but that number is set to sky rocket over the next few years as the population ages. By 2050, the number of people affected in the U.K. is expected to at least double and world-wide the figure is likely to reach 106 million with most of this increase being in the west and developed nations.

The disease itself is a chronic and progressing degenerative condition that affects the nervous system. These abnormal changes in the brain worsen over time until they can eventually interfere with nearly all of its functions. Usually starting with memory there is a gradual decline in other cognitive or thinking abilities and changes in personality and behaviour may then start to follow. This progression may take between 5 and 20 years, but once widespread loss of mental abilities occurs then very often the sufferer becomes totally dependant on others for their care and support.

It is not only these changes that take place within the sufferer that make this such a traumatic disease but the stress on the spouses, family and friends who need to provide the support that makes it so emotionally and physically draining as well.

Therefore it is not only for the sake of the sufferer but also for the carer that the information in this book is so vitally important.

The Early Warning Signs And Symptoms Of Alzheimer's Disease

There are a few tell-tale early warning signs to look out for with Alzheimer's disease and like any other condition early recognition can lead to an early diagnosis and treatment. Like any other condition, it is worth bearing in mind that an accurate diagnosis and treatment plan is not based on the presence of one or two of these signs but on the appearance of several. It is also important to note that there are normal variations and the degree to which any of these signs is present is important so as to differentiate it from the normal ageing process.

So, with that in mind, I will list some of the important signs to look out for whilst making a side note on any normal variations. The following list is not in any order of appearance (as signs may occur simultaneously or even come and go before becoming more permanent) it is just written in a way that can show you the progression of the condition.

1. The first major sign to look out for and be aware of is memory loss. Now this isn't the normal forgetting where you have put your keys, someone's name or even the occasional appointment, this is an increasing forgetfulness especially when it involves recently learned information. It may also lead on to misplacing items or putting them in inappropriate places – such as car keys in the refrigerator or the washing in the oven.

2. This memory loss may develop into problems with problem solving or abstract thinking. This is different to working out a shopping bill or balancing a cheque book and becomes difficulty with performing tasks and forgetting what objects are and how they should be used.

3. This may lead on to problems with language and word usage. Often people with Alzheimer's will forget simple words or substitute another incorrect word making their speech and writing difficult to follow. This is not when you occasionally forget a word or call something a "thingamajig" it is more when you talk about "that thing that I use on my head to keep my hair neat" instead of asking for the hair brush.

4. We have all gone into a room, forgotten why we went into it, had to retrace our steps and re-enter it – this is normal and a sign of a busy (forgetful) mind. However, difficulties may arise with Alzheimer's sufferers in performing familiar tasks and routines where they forget how to play games, prepare meals or use simple machines (like the washing machine or telephone).

5. I often forget which day of the week it is (they all seem to pass so quickly nowadays!) and occasionally I have arrived at a destination and wondered how I got there. With Alzheimer's, people can forget their own environment and neighbourhood and not know where they are, how they got there or why they are there.

6. There may be changes in mood and personality associated with the illness. This may range from mood swings such as becoming agitated, anxious, angry or tearful to just lethargic having lost the incentive to be actively involved (especially in conversation), just sitting in front of the television, sleeping and becoming more dependant on others. Although moods and personalities change as we age (they call it being cantankerous!) these moods are more extreme and changeable than normal and the failing to interact differs from tiredness and fatigue.

7. Acting inappropriately such as wearing the wrong clothes for the weather or season (or even too many sets of the same clothes) can be a warning sign. Also making inappropriate comments, gestures and actions may also be indicative of changes. These are more extreme than the occasional wrong decision or questionable comment that we may make during the course of a normal week.

Alzheimer's Disease:
Possible Causes and Risk Increasing Factors

Unfortunately, although there are no definitive causes for why some people develop Alzheimer's disease there are theories as to its cause, and there seems to be certain factors (or risk factors) that seem to increase the likelihood of someone developing the condition.

In this section I will cover the most common and most highly regarded theories and risk factors, because once it is known what may cause a specific problem action can be taken to counteract the steps that lead to it.

It would be nice to think that the solution could be easy – after all there are only two main causes that are recognised as being at the root of Alzheimer's (and most of the other dementias) and these are the result of either;

1, a loss of communication between the nerves of the brain and,
2, destruction of these nerves.

However, it isn't quite that simple!

There are several factors that may develop into these two causes and I will briefly discuss the theories behind them now.

The Theories Behind The Disease

For the sake of simplicity I have tried to link together the possible causes of Alzheimer's into categories. I personally believe that Alzheimer's is a multi-factorial (i.e. there is not one sole cause that leads to its development or progression) and I do not believe that there are any particular factors that are more likely to lead to its development. I feel it is the result of a combination of smaller dysfunctions and problems that build up to lead to the final end result. I have listed these categories in no particular order as, I believe, in their own small way they are all equally responsible.

1. Chemical Factors.

The cells and the nerves of the brain need to be able to communicate and talk to each other in order to fully function and they do this via neurotransmitters or chemical messengers. Anything that can hinder the action of these messengers will therefore have a detrimental effect on the functioning of the brain.

Studies of Alzheimer's sufferers have shown that they have lower levels of various neurotransmitters that are believed to influence intellectual functioning and behaviour. The cause of these lower levels may be reduced production or something that blocks their action. Both causes may be due to either chemical imbalances or increased toxicity from an outside source (such as heavy metals or homocysteine – which I will cover later).

2. Vascular disturbances.

A poor blood supply to the brain may also be a causative factor. This may be due to a diminished supply caused by ageing or through injury such as stroke or direct head trauma. Studies have shown, for example, that there is an increased risk of dementia and other neurological conditions amongst ex boxers (who seem to be prone to having their heads hit!).

3. Pre-existing conditions.

Illnesses such as diabetes, high blood pressure and high cholesterol have all been linked as causes of Alzheimer's disease. Studies show that high and uncontrolled blood pressure decreases the blood supply to the brain. Other studies have shown that almost three quarters of people who die of heart disease have amyloid plaques (which I cover further in point 9) in their brains typical of Alzheimer's sufferers.

4. Genetic Predisposition.

There have been two genetic / hereditary factors found that predispose a person to Alzheimer's (particularly early onset Alzheimer's disease) and these are either suffering from Down's Syndrome (a genetic defect) or a family history of dementia (a genetic / hereditary condition) as it seems there is a slightly higher risk of developing the condition if a first degree blood relative (parent / brother / sister) has developed it previously.

Researchers have linked at least ten percent of late onset Alzheimer's to the inheritance of a gene mutation (on chromosome 14) that directs production of apolipoprotein (ApoE) – a cholesterol carrying protein. There have also been other genetic mutations identified that may account for a predisposition to Alzheimer's and these occur on chromosomes 1, 12, 19 and 21.

5. Slow acting infections.

A slow-acting virus has been identified as a cause of some brain disorders that closely resemble Alzheimer's. These infections may precede the onset of Alzheimer's by many years and create an inflammatory process that damages the brain predisposing it to disease and deterioration.

6. Autoimmune diseases.

Autoimmune diseases may trigger a response that causes the body's normally protective immune system to begin to attack itself by producing antibodies which destroy its own cells.

7. Inflammatory conditions.

This is similar to the infection based theory in that researchers believe that Alzheimer's disease may result from an inflammatory process that creates abnormal waste products out of normal molecules and these may then attack healthy brain tissue. There seems to be some basis for this theory as researchers have found that anti-inflammatory medication (such as non-steroidal anti-inflammatories) seems to reduce the risk of developing the disease and also slow the rate of its progression.

8. The Tau Theory.

Another major theory behind the cause of Alzheimer's lays the blame on tau. Tau is a protein whose role is to act like the backbone or skeleton of a cell and organise and stabilise its shape and function. Unfortunately, during the progression of Alzheimer's the tau protein deforms and loses it's ability to offer support to the cell and it eventually aggregates and creates a tangle of nerve fibres. These aggregations are another hallmark of the progression of Alzheimer's disease.

9. The Amyloid Hypothesis.

This is the theory that seems to have the largest support. Amyloid precursor protein is a protein that is found throughout the body (although its function remains unclear) but in Alzheimer's disease there is a malfunction in the processing of it which leads to the formation of a protein "beta amyloid" fragment. These fragments slowly aggregate or clump together to form the amyloid plaques that are characteristic of the disease. These clumps then progress and build to cause nerve disruption and destruction.

10. Disruption in the manufacture of nerve growth factors

Another theory (that is gaining ground in areas of stroke, Alzheimer's and spinal nerve damage) is that there may be a disruption in either the manufacture or processing of so called nerve growth factors. These "nerve growth factors" are usually proteins whose job it is to regulate and control nerve cell repair, survival and maturation.

Now that I have covered the major theories that are believed to lead to the progression of Alzheimer's disease, I feel that it is important to look at the possible aggravating or risk factors that are associated with its development. Once we understand the possible causes and risks that are associated with the condition we are better prepared to tackle it – which we will do in sections two – six.

Risk Factors Associated With The Development Of Alzheimer's Disease.

As with the many theories behind the cause of Alzheimer's disease no one is certain as to why some people are more prone to the condition. Because of this there have been several key risk factors identified that may lead to it development and progression.

These are again listed in no particular order as no one factor is the major cause, but all are important.

1. Age

Alzheimer's is rare below the age of 65 but the chances of developing the condition increases dramatically as one gets older. Although less than 5% of the population will suffer with the disease before the age of 75, at age 85 or over this percentage rises to almost 50%.

Unfortunately, as the population not only ages but is expected to live longer this means that the number of cases can only increase.

2. Gender

It would appear statistically that women are more likely than men to develop the disease. This may be due to the fact that they have a longer life expectancy or it may be due to the fact that these figures are taken from residential home occupancy.

Without wanting to appear sexist (and this is an idea thought of by the World Health Organisation so blame them if you don't agree with it) if a married couple were to live into old age together and one of them were to develop the condition, it is more likely that if it were the man the wife would be more able to cope with him at home than if it were the wife and the husband had to manage and care for them both.

Therefore if it were the wife who develops the illness she is more likely to be cared for in a home as the husband is less able to manage – hence the figures increase for females patients with the illness in residential homes.

One factor that does have a direct link to gender is the role that the sex hormones (in particular oestrogen and Hormone Replacement Therapy) have in either developing or protecting against Alzheimer's. Research is unclear as to whether HRT may lead to the development of Alzheimer's or help protect against it. Early studies from the 1980's and 1990's seemed to indicate that it played a protective role, however the massive Women's Health Initiative Memory Study indicated that there was an increased risk of dementia in women taking oestrogen after the age of 65.

3. Lifestyle Factors.

As I touched upon earlier there are several lifestyle factors that can increase your chance of developing Alzheimer's disease. These include anything that affects your cardiovascular health (such as high blood pressure and cholesterol) but also poorly controlled diabetes and diet may be contributing causes.

Also included are factors such as whether you smoke, your exercise habits (both physical and mental) and the amount of alcohol you consume – both too little and too much are aggravating factors.

Another factor that can also be included in this section on lifestyle factors are direct exposure to toxins and heavy metals.

As I mentioned earlier in the section on chemical factors it has been believed for a long time that exposure to the heavy metals aluminium, mercury, copper or zinc may increase the likelihood of developing the condition.

4. Level of Education.

Some researchers have suggested that those with higher education are at a lower risk for Alzheimer's disease than those with less education. Although this has been repeatedly demonstrated in several studies the reason for this is unknown however it is believed that the more you use your brain the more nerve pathways and synapses (or brain connections) you make. The greater the numbers of these pathways you have the greater the reserve you have to fall back on if some of these pathways deteriorate. It may also be that the higher the level of education a person has the more they are able to hide or disguise the affects of the condition in its early stages.

5. Genetic predisposition

As I covered earlier there seems to be certain genetic and hereditary factors that increase the likelihood of developing Alzheimer's disease. These are certain chromosomal or genetic mutations and having a close blood relation that has already developed the condition.

6. Location.

It seems that there may be a distinct east / west divide when it comes to the prevalence of Alzheimer's in society. Research seems to indicate that there is a higher prevalence in urban rather than rural societies and that there is a greater incidence in the west rather than the east. Various studies show that the number of cases of Alzheimer's disease in Asia, India and Africa is lower than that reported from studies in developed countries such as the United States of America and Europe but the reasons for this are unclear. Many researchers believe that this variance may be purely due to differences in reporting the condition and the possibility that it may be called other things in other areas and societies reduces the number of cases identified.

Having covered the risk factors and theories behind Alzheimer's disease I would like to make it clear that at this stage it is impossible to predict exactly who may develop the condition. It must be remembered that it can strike anyone irrespective of age, gender, culture or class and therefore with that in mind it is time to move onto how the illness is handled from a medical viewpoint.

Medical Testing and the Diagnosis of Alzheimer's Disease

As with all conditions and illnesses, the earlier a diagnosis can be made the more likely it is that the prescribed treatment will be effective (the majority of the current medications for the treatment of Alzheimer's disease work best with an early diagnosis). Unfortunately, for those suffering with Alzheimer's at the moment there is no single test that can be used with 100% reliability. Therefore to improve the accuracy of diagnosis your medical practitioner will most probably prescribe a series of tests and procedures to give the most likely diagnosis.

[Alzheimer's disease can only be diagnosed with 100% accuracy after death as it is only then that the actual brain tissue can be examined at autopsy. With this in mind the best that medical doctors can do before that is to give a diagnosis of possible Alzheimer's where all the other causes have been ruled out or probable Alzheimer's where most of the other causes have been ruled out].

The following is a list of the various tests and screenings that may be carried out in order to rule out other diseases and illnesses and give the most likely (and accurate) diagnosis. When the following tests are performed (or those your medical doctor feels will be most valid) a diagnostic accuracy of between 80 - 90% can be established.

1. Firstly, an accurate medical history will be taken. This will either be a face to face consultation and / or a questionnaire, such as the Mini-Mental State Exam (or MMSE) or the 6 Item Cognitive Impairment Test (6CIT) to establish if there are any other underlying medical conditions that may be at the root of the changes and to help rule out other causes of depression or cognitive impairment. These tests will assess problem solving (such as performing simple calculations in your head), memory,

attention and hand-eye coordination. It will also assess any medications currently being taken, diet, lifestyle, alcohol consumption and which (if any) activities of daily living are being affected. It may also involved speaking with and questioning close family members.

These interviews and the diagnostic mental tests have been shown to have an accuracy of 89% when diagnosing Alzheimer's in the early stages – so these alone can give a pretty good indication of diagnosis.

2. A standard medical examination will follow that will check the heart (blood pressure and pulses) and lungs, as well as hearing and sight. Neurological tests such as checking reflexes, coordination and balance, muscle strength and tone may also be carried out. Simple laboratory tests that check blood and urine to rule out illnesses such as diabetes, thyroid or liver problems may be performed. In certain cases the cerebrospinal fluid (CSF) may be examined

3. Brain scans may be taken and these will either be CT scans, MRIs or PET scans to rule out the possibility of strokes, blood clots or tumours.

Several studies have confirmed the clinical accuracy of brain scans in the diagnosis of Alzheimer's although more research needs to be carried out especially using MRI and PET scans. PET scans are used to highlight areas in the body that metabolise glucose (the main source of fuel for the brain) and can pinpoint specific regions with a high or low glucose turnover.

Studies have shown that people with the APOE-e 4 gene (indicative of those that may eventually develop Alzheimer's disease) have reduced glucose metabolism in certain areas of the brain and these studies indicate that the lower the glucose metabolism in these areas the greater the cognitive decline at a later date.

Studies have shown that MRIs (which are used much more often) can detect brain deterioration and cellular loss at an even earlier stage in those people that later go on to develop Alzheimer's. A newer technique called dynamic MRI is now being developed in order to chart the deterioration and progression of the condition but this is less useful for diagnosis.

In addition to these standard tests for detecting Alzheimer's disease research is continually developing new approaches that may be beneficial in the early diagnoses of the condition. Some of these are:

1. Researchers at the Institute of Psychiatry at King's College London have identified certain proteins that can be detected in the blood of those diagnosed with Alzheimer's. They believe that when these proteins are found in higher than normal concentrations it may provide an early indication on the likelihood of developing the condition.

2. A team of researchers from the University of Pittsburgh and a separate team from UCLA have developed a molecule that sticks to beta-amyloid plaques (which are indicative of Alzheimer's) yet will no effect on normal

brain tissue. Using scanning techniques such as PET scans they can then look for this marker in the brains of those suspected of suffering cognitive decline and detect any early changes.

3. Researchers at the Mayo Clinic have noted a weight loss "trend" amongst women that later go on to develop Alzheimer's. Women that develop dementia tend to steadily loss weight (for no apparent reason) several years (and in a few cases up to a decade) before the first symptoms of Alzheimer's appear.

4. Researchers in the United States have held promising trials that indicate with an 80% accuracy that an electroencephalogram (EEG) test (where the nerves of the brain are tested electrically) can clearly demonstrate that the brains of those suffering from Alzheimer's react differently than those of healthy people.

5. Studies at the University of Columbia have shown that the inability to identify common smells may be indicative of Alzheimer's disease. The research has narrowed the smells down to a list of ten that seem to be predictive of early cognitive decline when sufferer is unable to identify eight or less. The list of smells is Clove, Leather, Lemon, Lilac, Menthol, Natural Gas, Pineapple, Smoke, Soap and Strawberry.

Alzheimer's Disease – The Medical Route

Before we investigate the many natural ways to slow and prevent the progression of Alzheimer's disease it is important to look at the medical options that may be available or that you may already be following. This is important for two reasons:

1. So that you can compare these with the alternatives, and

2. Sometimes the medical and prescription route is necessary particularly in severe cases where there may be changes in mood or personality.

This second point is important as people with dementia or suffering from Alzheimer's may at some stage of its progression develop symptoms such as depression, restlessness, aggressive behaviour and occasionally delusions and hallucinations. It is therefore important to not only understand the reasons for this behaviour but to effectively treat it – with prescribed medication if necessary.

Before we continue I must point out that as a practitioner of complementary therapies I always try to resort to medication as the last approach and, with that in mind, I would like to stress the following points.

1. Before any drugs are prescribed it is essential to ensure that the person with dementia is physically healthy, comfortable and well cared for. If, wherever possible, they are encouraged to live an active, near normal a life as possible (that has stimulating or interesting daily activities) it may be possible to avoid the use of drugs altogether. The less stress, distress or agitation a sufferer encounters the more routine their life may remain.

For example, often excessive or loud noises can worsen the agitation felt by individuals suffering with Alzheimer's. Simple steps that can create a calmer environment are using pleasant, simple activities to distract the individual, looking at old photos or memorabilia or listening to either soothing or their favourite music may all help to reduce or even eliminate the behaviour.

Hard as it can sometimes be if the carer becomes angry or frustrated in response to a difficult behaviour this only tends to upset the person with Alzheimer's and increases the severity of the behaviour and its frequency. Responding with a more calm, controlled manner can reduce the tension long enough to distract the individual so that the moment passes.

2. All drugs have side-effects which may worsen symptoms and the benefits of prescribed medication in these circumstances needs to be carefully weighed up before hand.

3. With any long term illness the body's natural chemistry (and especially that of the brain) will change and a drug that had initial benefits may no longer be as effective.

4. Always remember that certain drugs taken in combination may counteract each other. Therefore it is important to ask your doctor what medication is being prescribed, why it is being prescribed and if there are any known side-effects. Always remind him / her what other medications you are taking.

Also once you have started a course of medication it is also of value to remember these other points:

1. Any medication works most effectively when taken as prescribed. For these reasons it is important to take the right dose, at the right time of day and make a note of whether they should be taken with or without food.

2. Despite all the advances in medicine there are very few wonder drugs. For this reason it is important to remember that you may not see immediate results. Often (and this is especially the case with anti-depressants or mood altering medication) the benefits of the drug may take several weeks to appear.

3. Once you have started following your prescribed course of treatment it is important that it is reviewed regularly. Also make sure that all of you consultants, doctors, nurses and carers are aware of all the medications that you are taking.

4. Finally, make sure that all your medications are kept safely and securely stored away whilst you are not taking them.

I will cover some of the important medications for treating Alzheimer's and other dementias before going on to show you what you can do to help yourself and those that you may be caring for.

Drugs To Help Control Dementia

There is a lot of ongoing work at the moment into a new type of medication to block the effect of cholinesterase – a naturally occurring compound that depletes the brain of one of its essential neurotransmitters.

These drugs were originally developed to improve memory and the ability to carry out a normal life by increasing the amount of acetylcholine in the brain (which is a chemical that has a profound effect on learning and memory). They have also been shown to have a profound effect on many behavioural symptoms such as mood, apathy and over-all confidence. Because of this these drugs may lessen the need for other medications to control these symptoms (although care must be taken that higher doses do not cause insomnia and further increase agitation).

These drugs are usually the first line of treatment for those suffering Alzheimer's and are often used at the appearance of the first confirmed symptoms. They are used mainly in mild to moderate Alzheimer's disease and have been shown to postpone the worsening of symptoms from anything from 6 months to a year.

The drugs that fall into this category are:

Donepezil (Aricept)
Rivastigmine (Exelon)
Tacrine (Cognex)
Galantamine (Reminyl or Razadyne)

Aricept

Aricept is one of the most widely used drugs to treat the symptoms of mild, moderate and severe Alzheimer's disease. In about 50% of those that take Aricept it can help to prevent the progression of the condition for up to 12 months – in some of these cases the improvement may be marginal but a few patients that have received the medication have noted dramatic improvements.

Usually the dosage is started at a low level of about 5mg a day and if after a month or so this is being well tolerated the level may be further increased. This will depend on the affect that it is having on the condition but also on whether or not any side-effects develop. Although these may be minimal (as it is usually well tolerated by most users) they may include feelings of nausea, diarrhoea (or increased frequency of bowel movements), vomiting, bruising, sleep disturbance, muscle cramps, loss of appetite and fatigue.

Advise your doctor if you (or the person you are caring for) are currently taking any other medication as caution needs to be taken if the sufferer is also using non-steroidal anti-inflammatory medications (such as ibuprofen or aspirin) as these may further increase the risk of developing stomach problems and ulcers. Occasionally, Aricept has been known to cause tachycardia or a speeding up of the heart.

Exelon

Exelon is another commonly used medication for mild to moderate Alzheimer's as well as dementia that may result through Parkinson's disease. Similar in action to Aricept it may help to delay the progression of these conditions by up to 12 months with improvements ranging from marginal in the majority of cases to profound in the occasional few.

Exelon is prescribed in three formats – either as a capsule, liquid or patch and the dosages vary accordingly. With the capsule or liquid form it is usual to start with 1.5 mg twice a day increasing with tolerance up to 6mg twice a day over a few weeks, whilst the patch provides a dose of approximately 4.5mg initially building to 9.5mg a day over time.

With Exelon the side-effects are more pronounced with patients that weigh the least (and if weight loss is progressive it may need to be stopped) and these are usually stomach and bowel related, muscle weakness and fatigue, dizziness or drowsiness.

Again, care must be taken if already on anti-inflammatory medication, anticholinergic drugs (such as those used to treat depression or psychosis) or if suffering from lung or bladder problems, stomach or heart disease or if there is a history of seizures.

Tacrine

Tacrine has two beneficial roles in the treatment of Alzheimer's disease but it also has many side-effects that have led to the reduction in the number of people to which it is prescribed.

But to start with the good news...

Firstly, Tacrine reduces the depletion of acetylcholine (by inhibiting the action of the chemical that breaks down this neurotransmitter) which has many benefits in improving cognition and memory. Secondly, it increases the blood flow to the brain (especially the cerebral cortex – the part of the brain that helps to regulate emotions) and thorough both of these actions it may improve the memory in some Alzheimer's sufferers. Tacrine has to be taken for a few weeks before the effects are noticed and it is usually prescribed in capsule form, taken four times a day on an empty stomach (one hour before or two hours after a meal).

However, there are a few quite severe side-effects and precautions linked with Tacrine which means that it is not suitable for everyone and it is because of these that your medical doctor may be reluctant to prescribe it.

You must inform your medical doctor (and pharmacist) what other prescription drugs and vitamins you are taking as some of these may react with Tacrine. For example, certain atropine type drugs, cold, sinus and allergy medications, anti-inflammatory or ulcer medications will have an effect on its action. Also, a history of ulcers, heart, kidney, lung, urinary tract or liver disease will prevent it being prescribed as Tacrine has been known to cause liver damage.

As well as these contra-indications to its use, Tacrine can also cause the usual stomach problems (associated with similar medications in its class), loss of balance, drowsiness, fatigue, headache, muscle aches, rashes and changes in the skin or eye colour.

Reminyl and Razadyne

Both of these are forms of galantamine and are effective for mild to moderate Alzheimer's. Both are manufactured in tablet form with an initial dose starting at 4mg twice a day building to 12mg twice a day depending on how well the drug is tolerated - it is usually well tolerated and any side effects such as increased bowel movement, loss of appetite or weight loss are usually temporary.

Like the other medications in this group, care needs to taken if you are already being prescribed anti-inflammatory medication or certain antidepressants as they can make these drugs harder to metabolise. Occasionally these drugs may cause a slowing of the heart rate or bradycardia.

A few other drugs are also used in the treatment of Alzheimer's and these work in a slightly different way by regulating the activity of glutamate in the brain.

Glutamate is a substance that plays a key role in both memory and learning – however excessive amounts are neurotoxic which means that they disrupt the communication between the cells of the brain and may even cause them to die. One of the medications for treating the moderate to severe stages of Alzheimer's disease by this method is Namenda (memantine).

Namenda

Studies on the effectiveness of Namenda have shown that it can be successfully used (with worthwhile benefits) to slow the decline and deterioration in thinking and the ability to perform activities of daily living in sufferers with moderate to severe Alzheimer's disease. It has also been shown to work effectively with other Alzheimer's medication (such as the cholinesterase inhibitors that I covered earlier) and in theses cases the combined effects are enhanced.

The usual starting dose of Namenda is one 5mg tablet a day and this can increase over weekly intervals (depending on tolerance) to 15 mg a day. Unlike the other medications used in the treatment of Alzheimer's disease Namenda very rarely causes any gastrointestinal irritation and it's main side-effects are limited to headache, dizziness and confusion and it has fewer negative drug interactions like other medications used to treat this condition (although care must be taken with certain cold or flu medications).

It is common practice that as soon as confirmed signs of Alzheimer's disease are noted cholinesterase inhibitors are started as this is when they are most effective. When these are no longer proving to be beneficial their dosages may be tapered off and Namenda is introduced – and in certain circumstances both of these medications can be taken simultaneously.

The medications I have just covered are the main medications for dealing with the memory side of Alzheimer's disease, however there are other aspects of the condition that also need to be addressed as they are equally important and I shall quickly cover these now.

Other Medications You May Encounter

One of the major difficulties associated with all of the various dementias is that of mood swings or behavioural changes which may include agitation, depression, suspicion or anger. In these circumstances other drugs may be prescribed to deal with these changes. There are treatments available to treat aggression or agitation (anti-anxiety medications such as Ativan, BuSpar or Xanax), medications that may help with the associated paranoia, confusion or suspicion (anti-psychotic medications such as Risperdal and Zyprexa) and medication to treat any depression (antidepressants such as Pamelor, Paxil, Prozac and Zoloft).

As these medications all play an important role in the control of Alzheimer's related symptoms I will cover each of these three main groups in turn.

34

Anti-anxiety Medications

With most dementias there is often an anxiety state that accompanies the condition. These anxieties may manifest as panic attacks, fearfulness, phobias, irritation or nervousness. Whilst these states can be disturbing on there own, it is often the patient's demands for constant attention, company or reassurance that causes the greatest problem.

In these situations, a group of drugs known as benzodiazepines (such as Ativan, BuSpar or Xanax) are often recommended as they are quick acting – with improvements noticed usually within a few days and in a few cases within hours, and they tend to have few or less severe side-effects.

As with all medications the dosage and duration of time that the medication is taken for will be closely monitored by your doctor as their action will vary between individuals. Most patients will be prescribed a dose that increases over a period of time until the required results are obtained and this may result in medication being prescribed once, twice or even three times a day depending on the severity of the condition and the patient's chemical make up.

Side-effects that are commonly associated with these medications are sedation, fatigue, unsteadiness (including an increased tendency to fall) and unfortunately in a few cases they may even aggravate memory loss and confusion if this is already present.

Also there may be interactions with other medications that the patient may be already taking and it is vital that you inform you doctor of all medications (including over the counter medications) that are already being taken or prescribed.

For example, it is extremely important that alcohol should be avoided as the effects can lead to serious and possibly life threatening complications for when they are taken together, alcohol and any of the anti-anxiety medications depress the activity of the central nervous system. Other medications to be careful with because of possible interactions are antihistamines, muscle relaxants, sedatives, anticonvulsant, cardiac and certain pain medication.

One final note of caution is that sufferers taking anti-anxiety medications for a prolonged duration may develop a tolerance to, and /or a dependency on these drugs. For this reason the medication may be prescribed for short periods of time only unless the prescribing doctor feels that long term use is advisable.

Tranquillisers and Anti-psychotic Medications

Originally developed to treat schizophrenia, anti-psychotics (or neuroleptics) such as Risperdal and Zyprexa, are now frequently prescribed to those suffering with dementia to help reduce their agitation, sleep disturbances, aggression, delusions and loss of inhibitions (although their use in these cases remains controversial).

Like all medications side-effects can occur with these medications and although these may range from mild effects such as dizziness, sedation (which whilst reducing aggression and restlessness may aggravate confusion) or unsteadiness, they may progress to symptoms that mimic Parkinson's disease (with its associated slowness of movements, trembling and stiffness of the joints and limbs) and even death.

It is for this reason that the Committee on Safety of Medicines (CSM) has announced that two of the commonly used neuroleptic drugs Risperidone and Olanzapine (or Risperdal and Zyprexa as they are more commonly known) should no longer be prescribed for the treatment of behavioural symptoms in people with dementia. It also cautions against the use of other similar drugs, unless absolutely necessary, because there is an associated increase in mortality and a three times greater risk of stroke with those that take them.

Antidepressant Medication

Depression can be very common amongst those suffering with Alzheimer's disease and other forms of dementia and it may occur at any stage throughout the illness. Symptoms of depression can include a persistent low mood, mood swings and irritability – all of which can be effectively treated by antidepressants with improvements noticed usually within a matter of weeks.

Antidepressants (such as Pamelor, Paxil, Prozac and Zoloft) are usually prescribed over a longer time frame than the other medication that can be used to control mood and behaviour (often for periods of six months or more) and therefore it is important that they are taken regularly without missing doses.

Although they may take several weeks to become effective, side-effects if any can present after a couple of days. These are often minor (headaches, dizziness, dry mouth, nausea and blurred vision) and usually pass quickly. Variations of anti-depressants know as SSRI's (selective serotonin re-uptake inhibitors) are usually better tolerated by older patients and therefore these are often the starting drug of choice in most cases of dementia.

Now that I have covered the medical route or the path that is usually recommended by your general practitioner, it is now time to look at the alternatives that are available – and more importantly the things that you can do to help both yourself and your loved ones!

Section Two

Lifestyle and Mental Longevity

Before I go into detail on the various supplements, herbs and vitamins that you can take that will make dramatic improvements to your cogitative capabilities, slow down and even prevent dementia and Alzheimer's, I want to first cover some aspects of daily living that you can modify that will greatly reduce your own risks of mental decline.

Now, as a complementary therapist I am aware that a lot of people are reluctant to being pro-active in their own health care, instead preferring to delegate the responsibility to someone else, but a few minor tweaks is all that is necessary on your part to radically improve your own mind, thinking and retention.

All of the following lifestyle changes will make an improvement but of course you don't have to do them all – the choice is up to you. All I can tell you is that the more you implement the greater the effect you will have on your health, and the more you do the more they will work together with greater results. For example (and these figures are illustrative) if you make one small change you may make a 10% improvement, but if you make two changes instead of a 20% improvement the effects can be as great as 30-35%. To spur you on and encourage you that the more you for do yourself the better the results – I want to share with you a study that was presented in 2002.

Researchers from the University of Kuopio, Finland **(1)** studied and followed almost 1500 students over a 21 year period. During this time they compared the effects of three known risk factors in the development of Alzheimer's to see the results. The three factors they chose to study were the presence of the apolipoprotein E4 (ApoE) gene (which I discussed earlier as being the gene linked to the greatest risk of developing Alzheimer's – in roughly tripling your chance of developing the disease), high blood pressure and high cholesterol.

The results and conclusions that they came to at the end of the study were startling. They discovered that the greatest risk of developing Alzheimer's disease fell with the groups that had the highest cholesterol and the highest blood pressure i.e. the two treatable factors! **What this means is that those subjects that were able to maintain their cholesterol levels and their blood pressure particularly in middle age** (developing high blood pressure in old age was not found to be a risk factor in the development of Alzheimer's) **were less likely to develop Alzheimer's disease even if they were genetically prone to it!**

So now I've got your attention, let us begin...

The best place to start with any health regime that you want to pay dividends in the future is, not unsurprisingly, in the present! For you to have many good years ahead you need to insure that you have a firm, solid foundation now so that you can build on it. Stephen Covey describes this in his motivational book "The Seven Habits of Highly Effective People" as starting with the end in mind – so that is what we shall do!

We need to make sure that your present day health is as good as possible in order to safeguard your future health and, with that in mind, I want to list a few areas that you may want to check up on to see how well you are doing.

The first thing is to maintain ideal blood sugar levels and if you are diabetic to make sure that this is as accurately controlled as possible.

A study in Archives of Neurology **(2)** shows that the incidence of Alzheimer's disease is greatly increased amongst diabetics and those with poor blood sugar control (these two conditions increase the chance of developing the condition by 65%). It also showed that other forms of impaired brain function are increased hastening the development of senile dementia by 44%. The reason for this increase is not yet clear but there have been many strong theories as to why this may be. Diabetes has been shown to disrupt the brain (and other cells) signalling for insulin which may lead to an increase in nerve enzymes that stimulate the build up of tau protein – a key mechanism in the early stages of Alzheimer's disease.

Dysglycaemia (or poorly controlled blood sugar) may also be involved in the development of nerve fibre tangles and the clumping of nerves inside the brain characteristic of the condition. Diabetes and poor blood sugar control also damages important blood vessel and their capillary networks increasing the risk of mini strokes or trans ischaemic attacks (TIAs) within the brain

Researchers at Northwestern University have now termed Alzheimer's disease as "type 3 diabetes" because of the effects of insulin on the brain. Insulin is vital for memory formation and cognition because when it binds to receptors within the nerves it triggers a mechanism for them to not only survive but form memories. However, a protein has been found in the brains of those suffering from Alzheimer's which removes insulin from these nerve cells, makes them insulin resistant and prevents them from firing properly **(3)**.

So, what do I recommend?

I would suggest a supplement of Chromium Picolinate is taken on a daily basis.

Various studies have indicated that chromium picolinate can have a significant effect on diabetes. Researchers have shown that it can help decrease insulin levels and improve blood sugar metabolism in both obese people and those with type 2 diabetes or other forms of impaired glucose tolerance.

Another important action of chromium is that it may also help prevent and reverse atherosclerosis and coronary artery disease (an area I will be covering shortly regarding its effects on dementia). This link is very strong as research has shown that those subjects with a chromium deficiency have elevated serum cholesterol and that once

it has been supplemented into their diets the level drops –
whilst increasing the level of HDL cholesterol (the "good"
cholesterol). Cardiologists have also noted that levels of
apolipoprotein B (APO B) one of the strongest predictors
of heart disease also drops dramatically.

Recommendation

A daily supplement of 200mcg of chromium
picolinate (or Chromium GTF) may be beneficial in
regulation blood sugar levels and the prevention of
atherosclerosis.

The next area to look into is maintaining a healthy
heart and circulation.

During a 10 year study of the elderly it was noted
that those who were mentally fit at the start of the study
and who later suffered a non fatal stroke were much more
likely to suffer from dementia or a decline in cognition
than those who had not. Unfortunately the study also
showed that if there were already signs of mild cognitive
impairment before the stroke then these signs were greatly
increased after the attack **(4)**. Another study **(5)** showed
that following a stroke cognitive and functional ability
declined significantly and behavioural scores decreased
modestly when compared against someone who had not
undergone a stroke.

What does this all mean?

Simply, that if you already have some form of decrease in your mental capabilities a stroke will make it far worse and if you didn't have any decrease before hand you stand a far greater chance of losing some mental capacity following a stroke.

This you may think (as I do!) is common sense. Loss of brain tissue through any means is likely to have some effect on how the brain works and as the brain ages and loses some of its ability to repair then this loss is going to be more greatly noticed.

So, what are the factors that have been most commonly found to affect circulation and therefore increase the chances of Alzheimer's disease?

Hypertension,
Diabetes – which I have already mentioned,
Hypercholesterolemia – increased cholesterol,
Hyperhomocysteinemia – high levels of homocysteine,
Atrial fibrillation – irregular heart beat and
Atherosclerosis – the build up of plaque inside blood vessels

We will look at these in turn, starting at the top of the list and as we work through them you will see how they are all connected and impact upon one another.

Hypertension or as it is more commonly known "high blood pressure" is a condition where blood pressure is raised over a long period of time. Although, it may have many causes ranging from stress and diet to kidney disease its effects can be devastating if left untreated. Persistent hypertension is one major cause of strokes, heart attacks, heart failure and aneurysm as well as being implicated in renal failure and a reduced life expectancy – all because the blood flows through the arteries with too much force. Even more importantly (with regards to this book) it is linked to cognitive decline, dementia and Alzheimer's disease.

A 15 year long study carried out in Sweden showed that vascular causes of dementia may be more common than we first thought **(6)**. Another study confirmed that elevated levels of blood pressure in middle age can increase the risk for late age dementia in men never treated for hypertension with anti-hypertensive medication **(7)**.

These two studies are significant in that originally it was thought that a high diastolic pressure (the lower figure) was the only risk factor but now a high systolic pressure (the upper figure) has also been implicated. Also earlier research was unclear as to the effects of treatment of blood pressure on Alzheimer's disease – some studies initially showed that there was a greater chance of developing Alzheimer's if your blood pressure had been medically treated – but now they are clearly coming out in favour of medically treating blood pressure to reduce the incidences of dementia in later life. One of the latest studies published in 2006 showed that medically treated hypertension may reduce the incidence of Alzheimer's disease by up to 70% in later life **(8)**.

Although the connection between blood pressure and dementia remains unclear recent studies have given light to two possible explanations. A recent study revealed that high blood pressure caused a reduced blood flow in the brains of Alzheimer's patients. This makes them even more susceptible to the effects of the disease by reducing the amount of oxygen that is supplied to the brain. Another study has shown that insulin (which has blood vessel dilation properties) resistance may be responsible for the increased arterial pressure in some patients with hypertension.

As you can see from the above – all the functions of the body are related. Therefore it is essential to control and maintain both your blood pressure and blood sugar levels if you are to lower your risk of developing Alzheimer's or dementia. Unfortunately there is a major drawback to the control of both of these and that comes from certain medications...

The May 2006 issue of Diabetes Care contained a study that shows how two types of high blood pressure medications may raise the risk of developing type 2 diabetes. The article relates to a study carried out by the Harvard Medical School comparing the incidence of hypertension drug use with diabetes statistics from nearly 75,000 subjects. The researchers found that thiazide diuretics increased diabetes risk by 36 percent in men, 20 percent in older women and 45 percent in younger women. Those that took beta-blocker drugs increased their diabetes risk by 20 percent increase for men and by more than 30 percent in older women.

Therefore it may be wiser to see if you can lower your blood pressure naturally and there are many supplements that can help you but, as a place to start, I would recommend the following.

One of the most beneficial natural treatments for hypertension is garlic. It not only helps reduce blood pressure, reduce triglycerides but also reduces the stickiness of the blood inside the arteries – thereby preventing the blood from clotting, which could otherwise cause a heart attack or stroke. I would recommend a supplement of 500mg of garlic three times a day (and a little parsley to reduce any unwanted breath or body odour!)

Another effective supplement for lowering high blood pressure is co-enzyme Q10 (CoQ10) – a natural substance produced in the body – as it can lower blood pressure almost as effectively as medication in some people without side effects. I would recommend a supplement of 100mg of co-enzyme Q10 daily.

Hawthorn also has proven heart benefits (especially amongst diabetics) and I would recommend a daily supplement of between 1000mg and 1200mg.

Recommendation

A daily supplement of 500mg three times a day of garlic may be beneficial in the treatment of hypertension.

A daily supplement of 100mg of co-enzyme Q10 may be beneficial in the treatment of hypertension.

A daily supplement of 1000mg to 1200 mg of hawthorn extract may be beneficial in the treatment of hypertension.

The next area to look at is hypercholesterolemia or high levels / increased blood cholesterol.

Researchers from the University of Kuopio, Finland (yes, it's that place again) teaming up with researchers from Kaiser Permanente Division of Research in Oakland, California have found that high cholesterol levels even as early as aged forty increase the risk of Alzheimer's disease by as much as one and a half times. Although researchers have known about the link between high cholesterol and Alzheimer's for many years it has been unclear as to the age at which lifestyle can start to affect dementia risk – and that is what makes this latest study more alarming.

The study **(9)** followed the health of almost 10,000 men and women in northern California from 1964 to 2007. The volunteers were aged between 40 and 45 when the study began. By 2007, around 500 had Alzheimer's and 162 had vascular dementia. Those with cholesterol levels between 249 and 500 milligrams in their 40s were one and a half times more likely to have Alzheimer's 40 years later than those with less than 198mg. People with levels of 221 to 248mg were more than one and a quarter times more likely to develop the disease.

The results of this latest study are important in that they show the risk of developing Alzheimer's disease due to high cholesterol is present regardless of whether patients suffered from other Alzheimer's-linked conditions such as diabetes, obesity or high blood pressure.

Maintaining a correct cholesterol level is important for two reasons. Firstly, it is believed that high cholesterol triggers the over-production of a protein that is improperly handled by those with Alzheimer's and this abnormal processing sets off a chain reaction that causes it to accumulate and build-up forming plaques that can kill brain cells. Also other research has shown that high cholesterol levels significantly increase the rate at which these tangles are formed **(10)**.

Secondly, the researchers concluded that high cholesterol also increases the production of a different protein that transports cholesterol out of the cell. Whilst that's a normal function, in this situation it results in an increase in free cholesterol which has a toxic effect on nerve cells **(11)**.

Unfortunately the jury is still out on the effects of taking statins with regards to the control of dementia and Alzheimer's disease. Several studies from 2000 showed there was a significant improvement in terms of lowered risks of dementia amongst those using statins to treat high cholesterol. One study showed a 60%-73% lower risk of developing the disease **(12)** whilst another showed that the risk of dementia was up to 70% lower for patients using statins compared with patients who had untreated high cholesterol or those receiving other lipid-lowering drugs **(13)**.

The rationale behind the effectiveness of statins is that Alzheimer's may be caused by poor blood flow and vascular changes in the brain, which statins may help to prevent. Also, researchers have found significantly fewer tangles in the brains of people who had taken statins than those who had not (even allowing for variables such as age, gender and past health).

However these studies considered a far smaller group of participants than a later study in 2005 which looked at almost 2800 subjects and found no reduced risk at all **(14)**.

Because of this uncertainty, we need to look at how to control and lower your cholesterol levels naturally – if they are high.

As a complementary therapist my first port of call would be vitamin E as this is known to have many beneficial effects on the body. With regards to cholesterol, vitamin E not only prevents but also removes atherosclerotic plaques (the fatty build up in artery walls) **(15)** but generally reduces "bad cholesterol" **(16)**.

Other studies have shown that vitamin E when combined with vitamin C offers an even greater protection against Alzheimer's, with one study stating that "the use of these antioxidant vitamins may offer an attractive strategy for the prevention of Alzheimer's disease" **(17)**. I would recommend a daily supplement of between 200-400i.u. of Vitamin E to safe-guard the integrity of the cardiovascular system

Another promising supplement is Arjuna. This is a herb that helps maintain a healthy heart by promoting effective cardiac functioning, regulates blood pressure, lowers cholesterol (by suppressing the blood's absorption of lipids) and reduces the effects of stress and nervousness. Studies have shown that it can effectively lower cholesterol by as much as 12 percent in just 30 days and therefore I would recommend a daily supplement of up to 250mg. of Arjuna.

Recommendation

A daily supplement of 200i.u. to 400 i.u. of vitamin E may be beneficial in the reduction of cholesterol.

A daily supplement of 250mg of Arjuna may be beneficial in the reduction of cholesterol.

Next on the list is hyperhomocysteinemia.

Hyperhomocysteinemia or high blood levels of homocysteine (a blood protein) is a relatively new area of investigation in the health field but it is rapidly becoming recognised as a major indicator of health.

It is appropriate that this section on homocysteine follows on from high cholesterol as homocysteine is an amino acid that actually increases the levels of bad cholesterol in the blood as well as damaging the lining of arteries and promoting blood clots. A study in the New England Journal of Medicine **(18)** shows that people who have high blood levels of homocysteine are the ones most likely to suffer Alzheimer's disease and a study from the Boston University School of Medicine revealed that a high homocysteine level can double your chance of developing either Alzheimer's or some other form of dementia.

Although homocysteine is necessary for several metabolic processes, excess amounts are toxic to the body and it is therefore critical to have the correct nutrition to prevent this toxic build up. Unfortunately it is estimated that over 75% of the population do not have an adequate diet to prevent this homocysteine overload.

The good news is that supplements of vitamins B6, B12 and folic acid, eating plenty of cereals and green leafy vegetables are extremely effective in helping to reduce your homocysteine level – and they are readily available from any health food or grocery store.

More impressive than the ease of which these vitamins are available are the studies that have shown that folic acid can cut homocysteine levels by about a fourth, and when combined with vitamin B12, homocysteine levels sank another 7%!

It is easy for a doctor to check your level of homocysteine to see just how high it is but as a general rule I would recommend that a good starting point for everyone is 1mg of folic acid building up to 5mg in severe cases of hyperhomocysteinemia, 50mg to 100mg of vitamin B6 (depending on severity) and 1mg of sub-lingual vitamin B12.

Another supplement that I would consider adding alongside those B vitamins is a substance called betaine.

Betaine is a nutrient that plays an important role in the health of the cardiovascular system and works closely with the B vitamins to break down and reduce the toxic levels of homocysteine. Studies have shown that homocysteine levels can drop by a factor of 40% in a number of weeks with a decrease being noted after the first day. Although 6 grams a day have been shown to be safe and have the most dramatic effects, I would recommend a supplement of 2 grams of Betaine HCl a day.

Recommendation

A daily supplement of 1mg to 5mg of folic acid may be beneficial in the reduction of homocysteine.

A daily supplement of 50mg to 100mg of vitamin B6 may be beneficial in the reduction of homocysteine.

A daily supplement of 1mg of sub-lingual vitamin B12 may be beneficial in the reduction of homocysteine.

A daily supplement of 2g of Betaine HCl may be beneficial in the reduction of homocysteine.

Now I would like to turn our attention to atrial fibrillation.

Atrial fibrillation is one of the main types of cardiac arrhythmia – or abnormal heart rate or rhythm. Atrial fibrillation causes a rapid and irregular heartbeat, during which the upper two chambers of the heart that receive blood (the atria) quiver or "fibrillate" instead of beating normally. Because of this irregular beating the heart cannot pump blood away from itself efficiently and therefore blood tends to collect and pool in the heart increasing the risk of clotting. These clots can then travel the body in the blood supply and may become lodged elsewhere causing strokes or pulmonary embolisms.

Unfortunately research published in the November 6th 2007 issue of Neurology (19) has also shown that the rate of dementia and Alzheimer's disease may progress more rapidly in those people suffering with atrial fibrillation – and they believe that by treating this condition it may actually slow or prevent the onset of Alzheimer's. In fact the research showed that atrial fibrillation may increase the rate of progression of Alzheimer's disease by up to 75%.

The lead researcher in the study reported that "the possibility that specific vascular conditions may affect how fast a person with Alzheimer's disease declines provides new opportunities for slowing the rate of Alzheimer's progression. Treatments for atrial fibrillation (and high blood pressure) are relatively inexpensive and safe and may reduce memory decline in Alzheimer's disease patients with these conditions."

There several types of medication and, if necessary, surgical interventions available in the treatment of atrial fibrillation but there are several common-sense approaches that you can also undertake to minimise your risk of getting atrial fibrillation or reduce the severity of it should you already suffer from the condition.

These steps are to:

1. Control your cholesterol and high blood pressure.
2. Maintain your correct blood sugar levels and control your diabetes.
3. Do not drink more than two alcoholic drinks per day.

4. Stop smoking.
5. Control your weight and / or lose weight if necessary, and
6. Get regular exercise – 20-30 minutes 2-3 times a week.

To finish this section on how the heart and its contributing factors may increase your risks of developing Alzheimer's and dementia, I will briefly cover the effects of atherosclerosis as several studies have found links with this, high cholesterol and the presence of apolipoprotein E – both of which I have mentioned before.

A study in published in the Lancet in 1997 **(20)** showed that there was a dramatic increase in the rate of all dementias when atherosclerosis was present and that the risk of developing any of the forms of dementia increased with the increasing levels of it. This study also high-lighted that the adverse effects of atherosclerosis when considering the development of Alzheimer's disease and vascular dementia were further increased by the presence of apolipoprotein E.

An additional study published in 2003 **(21)** added further weight to this study when it revealed that there was an association between severe atherosclerosis in the brain and sporadic Alzheimer's and that this should be considered a risk factor for this dementia. These observations strongly suggest that atherosclerosis-induced brain hypoperfusion (or decreased blood flood which, if prolonged, may result in permanent cell dysfunction and death) contributes to the clinical and pathological manifestations of Alzheimer's disease.

To lower the risks of atherosclerosis I would recommend following the 6 lifestyle changes already described as well as increasing the amount of oats and barley that you consume in you diet (easily achieved by changing your breakfast cereals) and supplementing with garlic (which I have already discussed).

Recommendation

A supplement of 150 grams of whole oat products and 30 grams of barley bran a day may help lower your risk of atherosclerosis and reduce you total cholesterol (and bad cholesterol) in particular.

The next two areas of lifestyle changes that we need to address are those of both physical and mental fitness.

The Affects of Physical Exercise on Alzheimer's Disease and Dementia

Being over weight and in particular being obese (determined either by a Body Mass Index of over 30 for adults or else looking in the mirror and asking yourself "Do I look too large" and answering truthfully!) can dramatically increase the risk of all types of dementia and Alzheimer's. In fact, a review of the literature shows that the increase can be almost two times as great.

Unfortunately, the news gets even worse...

Further research published in the journal Neurology **(22)** has shown that those subjects (out of a sample of 6,500) that measured the greatest increase in abdomen size over the 30 years of the trial were more than **three times** as likely to develop dementia. This was irrespective of whether or not their weight had increased – they just had to have developed larger bellies.

The reasons behind this aren't clear but it may be related to the fact that increased abdominal fat is also linked to diabetes, heart disease, increased blood pressure and strokes – all of which have a direct correlation with the increased incidence of Alzheimer's disease and dementia.

So what are the two best ways to avoid weight gain and increased abdominal fat? I believe the two best ways are exercise and diet which we will cover in detail later in the book, but before I do it is worth re-iterating and certainly worth remembering that what it is good for the heart is also good for the head!

The good news is that the exercise involved or the amount of time spent exercising does not have to be too strenuous or too long. Also, research has shown that the more frail a person is before they begin an exercise regime the more that exercise was likely to help them. This means that the exercise you partake in doesn't have to be too physical, too time consuming and best of all if you are in poor shape to start with (both physically and mentally) it will still have an effect!

Research has shown **(23)** that 15 minutes of exercise, three times a week ranging from the following activities – walking, hiking, bicycling, aerobics or callisthenics, swimming, water aerobics, weight training or stretching was enough to slow down the rate of Alzheimer's disease or even delay it's onset by up to 40%! Another research paper states that it should even be considered as part of the treatment programme **(24)**.

As well as the affects that simple exercise can have on cognitive function it also has other positive benefits. These include reducing the severity of the depression that is often associated with dementia (some studies suggesting that up to 70% of patients with dementia may also suffer from depression), reducing the number of falls (a common problem amongst the elderly but one that is more common amongst Alzheimer's suffers) and reducing the amount of "aimless" wandering that is often associated with these conditions – as the sufferer becomes more engaged in time filling activities they are less prone to wander out of boredom. Another added benefit of regular exercise is that it can naturally improve sleep and sleeping habits (again fitful or disturbed sleep is common in those that suffer from Alzheimer's or other forms of dementia).

Exercise doesn't have to involve strenuous activity but it just has to get the blood pumping a little faster, increase the breathing rate and last at least 15-20 minutes, three times a week (and it can always be longer and harder should you so desire!).

Also, exercise (like people) comes in all shapes and sizes and should involve something you enjoy or something that needs doing. Cleaning is a good example of something that at least falls into the second category. Research has shown that those people that actively clean (and this includes sweeping, polishing, mopping, cleaning windows etc.) for 20 minutes at a time still had a respectable 20% decrease in the risk of developing Alzheimer's. It doesn't just have to be housework either; gardening and D.I.Y. also count towards the exercise stakes and this can include mowing the lawn, raking up leaves and moss, hedge trimming, pruning etc.

There are another couple of benefits with incorporating household chores into your exercise regime and the first is that there isn't any equipment to buy or a routine to learn – most of the equipment needed is found under your kitchen sink and the "moves" involved have usually been learnt by rote years ago. The other benefit is that the more elbow grease you exert the better it is with regards to memory improvement – and you can see the results of your hard efforts not only in your surroundings looking much better but also with noticeable improvements in joint mobility and general flexibility.

If you do decide to start up an exercise routine (and I would suggest that you seriously think about it) there are a few little pointers I would recommend. These are...

1. Don't eat anything heavy a couple of hours before vigorous exercise.

2. Make sure you drink plenty of fluids before, during, and after your workout – water is ideal.

3. Adjust your activity according to how you are feeling on that day and the weather – don't try to do to much if you don't feel up to it, you are tired or ill and don't over exert if it is too hot.

4. Listen to your body. If your exercise regime induces chest pain, irregular heartbeat, undue aches, pains or tiredness, nausea, unexpected breathlessness or light headedness stop what you are doing and if the feelings do not subside see your doctor.

5. Remember to have a warm-up and cool-down period.

The Affects of Mental Exercise
on Alzheimer's Disease and Dementia

The old adage of "use it or lose it" is very true with all parts of the body. We know that decreased exercise causes muscles to weaken and waste and bones to become brittle or osteoporotic – and the same is true for the brain!

I have already shown how the more education a person has the lower their risk of developing Alzheimer's disease and other dementias are. Some studies even suggest that the risk of Alzheimer's is increased by 2-4 times in those with a lower level of education **(25, 26)**. Before you start worrying that you were never any good at school and that you wish you had tried harder **the good news is it is never too late to make improvements!**

Various studies have shown that those people that participate in the most activities (particularly those that are mentally stimulating) have a lower incidence of Alzheimer's disease. Also, if a person is already suffering from dementia or Alzheimer's the more mentally and intellectually difficult and challenging the activities are the less they are likely to decline **(27, 28, 29)**.

There are many reasons for this and the real reason may be a combination of factors. The more exercise and mental stimulation you get may increase the blood flow to the brain and reduce the incidence or effects of vascular disease. The more the brain is mentally stimulated the more pathways it develops so that the effects of dementia or Alzheimer's disease may take longer to show. It is also believed that the more the brain is used the more it builds up a reserve or capacity (technically called a "cognitive reserve") and the longer it takes for this reserve to be diminished. But, whatever the reason the more the brain is used and stimulated the better it functions throughout later life.

The next few pages provide you with various ideas that you may find helpful in kick-starting your brain – and best of all most of them are enjoyable!

<u>Activities That Alzheimer's Sufferers Should / Could Be Involved With.</u>

One of the major problems faced by those suffering from Alzheimer's disease or any of the dementias is the periods of loneliness, boredom and frustration.

It is therefore important for both the sufferer and the carer that these "empty times" are as few and far between as possible. This not only gives the carer some respite (knowing that the person they are looking after is somewhat occupied) but also reduces the amount of time that the sufferer has trying to occupy himself in activities such as wandering.

When possible try to fill these empty times with activities that are creative, helpful and enriching but also those that are both physically and mentally rewarding.

The following list of ideas is not exhaustive and you may find that some of the activities are more applicable to your situation than others. You may also have favourite past-times of your own that you may wish to use and that's fine as every situation and case is unique. However, these ideas will give you a starting point in finding activities that will stimulate the mind, involve physical activity or that can just be used to occupy the odd moment.

Music and Films

Anything that involves music is particularly useful and easy to carry out. These may be activities that involve just listening to music and watching music videos / DVDs or musicals, to joining in and singing along to particularly older, well known songs.

It is possible to take the singing of songs further and incorporate it in to various games. These may include things such as "Name that Tune" where either a certain number of notes are played or lyrics sung and someone has to try and guess the song (and they can then complete it should they wish by singing the rest). A song title could be given that has a word missing and someone has to try to fill in the blank, or even you could try to name songs by certain artists and singers in a form of "who sung what".

Depending on the amount of dementia or past interests activities can also include playing musical instruments especially rhythm instruments (as a side note music therapy can be very beneficial with regards to some of the behavioural problems that are often associated with dementia), dancing or even playing a role in local or nursing home shows, productions and plays – as long as the role is not to taxing or over stimulating. If you feel this may be a little too much then it is possible to just to attend various shows, plays, pantomimes etc.

Films, television and DVDs can not only be nostalgic but also useful, informative and an aid to memory retention and cognition. By watching and discussing films it is possible to open up conversation and debate but also reminisce on past personal history and events. These topics may be former occupations (first job, pay etc.), past holidays or anniversaries, significant historical events of the time, great inventions or break-throughs, war related events – such as military service or work in other related organisations.

These discussions can then lead on to asking for advice and information regarding your own work or related events (even if the advice is not used the person giving it still feels involved and of use) and the discussions can be ever growing to even include help with every day activities.

Craft and Hobby Activities

Crafts and hobbies are an excellent way to not only produce something creative and of sentimental value but also keep the mind active, increase dexterity and also occupy some time for both the carer and the sufferer. Again, this list whilst not being exhaustive will give you some ideas of past-times that may be applicable to your own circumstances.

Playing cards is a good starting point for anyone suffering dementia as it can improve memory, hand – eye co-ordination, hand dexterity and be either a solo, paired or group activity. Solo games such as "Patience" can fill many an hour whilst paired and group games can range from simple memory games such as pairing the cards (or "Fish"), to "Snap" continuing up to bridge and poker depending on the ability and severity of the sufferer.

Also, it is worth thinking about crossword puzzles word searches, word association games, brainteasers, puzzles and memory exercises – there is an entire industry based now on "brain training" with various computer software available to keep the mind active. It may surprise you to realise that it was the work of Professor Kawashima in Kyoto that has led to the development of Nintendo's DS console for brain training.

The computer game is based on his research into Alzheimer's disease and how simple tasks that are performed on a daily basis actually improve mental functioning and conditioning over time. At one of Japan's memory loss clinic they actual give copies of his books and these games consoles to their patients to use at home!

One important thing to note is that for better results the games you choose to participate in must get harder as you go along. If you like cross-word puzzles make sure that the difficulty is increased over a period of time so that the mind is stretch and pushed to its ever increasing limits!

The following few pages gives you some ideas as to games and logical puzzles that are easy to implement and carry out. These ideas are from an excellent book called "What Your Doctor May Not Tell You About Alzheimer's Disease: The Complete Guide to Preventing, Treating, and Coping with Memory Loss" by Gayati Devi and Deborah Mitchell and it is well worth a read for other "brain boosting activities you may want to consider.

All of these activities require very little in the way of materials – just a pen, paper and a stopwatch or clock. What is better is that they can all be carried out at little or no cost and you should start to notice an improvement if you just invest 30 minutes of your time a couple of days per week.

Anagrams

On a piece of paper write down a long, polysyllabic word (like "paraphernalia") at the top of the page in bold – this is your starting point. Then write down as many words as you can make from this word in 15-20 minutes by moving the letters around. Try to make words that are at least three letters long (the longer the better) and you can include proper names (names of people, places, things) as well as foreign words – just don't make them up!

For example, "hernia", "nail", "pear", and "air" are words that can be made from "paraphernalia" when you rearrange the letters.

Here are some other polysyllabic words (and a few ideas as to words that you can make from them) to get you started:

Administration: station, mini, ration, mind
Autobiographical: auto, graph, photo, tool
Bacteriological: logical, bacteria, glacier, broil
Depolarization: polar, deport, ratio, trapezoid
Epidemiological: logical, mould, gloom, damp
Individualistic: dual, individual, vial, last
Participatory: party, tapioca, captor, tray
Rationalization: ration, nation, lion, riot
Sentimental: sentiment, mental, listen
Totalitarianism: total, talisman, militant, raisin

Categories

On your piece of paper, write the name of a specific category at the top. For example, "Wild Animals", "Boy's Names", "Sports" etc. and then for 15-20 minutes write down as many items as you can in that category.

If you get stuck after a while this is okay because it allows you to ask questions that can also be used a memory joggers. For example if you chose "Wild Animals" and you've listed twelve animals but can't think of any others try asking yourself the following questions for a little bit more stimulation....

- What types of animals have I seen at the zoo?
- What types of animals have I seen at a circus?
- Which animals live in Africa?
- Which animals have I ever seen while on vacation?
- Which animals do some people hunt?

Another way to jump-start your brain and "get those juices flowing" is to take each letter of the alphabet and think about which animal begins with that letter. For example if you chose the letter "A" you might say "aardvark", "anteater" or "antelope." For "B," you might list "bear", "buffalo," and "baboon".

Here are some other categories you can use for your sessions – but you can always pick others if nothing appeals to you, or you cannot think of any examples to fit the category – you can always come back to it later!

- Cars,
- Birds,
- Flowers,
- Trees,
- Countries,
- Types of dog / breeds,
- Girl's names,
- Mammals,
- Colours.

Word Associations

Make a list of five to ten nouns, one word to a line, down the left side of your paper, leaving several blank spaces between each word. Then list five words that are associated with each of the nouns.

For example, if one of the nouns you chose is "Polar Bear", you might list the following associated words: white, furry, Alaska, North Pole, animal.

It is easy to make a list of nouns (despite what you may be thinking) and to get you started here are some ways to get ideas:

- Look around you: what's in the room you're in? Perhaps there's a sofa, lamp, bookshelves, stereo or television? If you're outside there may be cars, trees, lamp posts, gardens or houses. So already we have ten words to get you started!

- Picture in your mind your favourite place to visit and list all the objects that you see. If you enjoy the beach then things that you may include might be sand dunes, seagulls, shells, umbrellas and waves.
- List five or ten gifts you would like to receive or give to someone else.
- List five foods in your refrigerator and five items in your bedroom closet.
- List five nouns that begin with "A" and five that begin with "B". You can continue at each session using two different letters of the alphabet for up to thirteen weeks!
- List five things you'd find in a grocery store and five things you'd find in a hardware store.

If this gets to easy then to stretch the imagination a little further you may wish to increase the number of nouns associated with each object. You could start with just five nouns and build up to ten or if that is still too easy challenge yourself and try to list even more.

Maths Works

This is a brain boosting exercise you can do whilst shopping. While in the store, mentally add up the cost of the items you put in your cart. Set a goal; say, you'll add up the cost of five items before you write down the total. Increase the number of items you add mentally each time you shop. Although this is mainly a maths exercise it also stimulates working memory.

Start with low-priced items (less than one pound if possible – although that is quite difficult these days): for example, 89 pence plus 59 pence equals £1.48 and continue adding more products. Once you can add up five items successfully in two or three trips, increase the number you add up mentally to six, then seven and so on.

Now, let's carry on with other ideas…

Board games can also be an ideal way to occupy and stimulate. Again the spectrum can range right the way through from games that require no skill (such as "Ludo" and "Snakes and Ladders") to "Dominoes", "Draughts", chess, trivia games where you can focus on areas or eras that the person knows best or that can recall the easiest (you can find questions from various trivia books, the internet or even making up your own questions) to "Pictionary" where someone has to draw an object for the others to guess.

Solo games can include "Jigsaw" puzzles which are again terrific for improving hand dexterity and co-ordination and are available in different levels of difficulty depending on the ability of the person they are aimed at.

Practical hobbies can include making cards by collecting pictures and photographs from various sources (or using other materials such as string, beads, glitter and so on) and this allows all year activities as the range of occasions suitable for these would be birthdays, anniversaries, holidays, Christmas, Easter, Valentines (always the romantic that I am!), get well soon cards, congratulations etc. Making scrap-books, photograph albums or collages of family occasions and holidays would also fit into this area.

The garden or yard also provides ideal opportunities for activities that are not too arduous. Starting a herb, flower or vegetable plot can provide physical and mental activity whilst giving a goal to aim for and a sense of achievement when they come to fruition. The produce can then lend itself to herb drying, flower pressing or flower arranging, preparing the vegetables or even cooking.

The garden or yard can also lend itself to the installation of bird tables, bird boxes or feeding trays all of which can be made quite easily (again involving everyone) from simple kits or materials that can be easily obtained. When installed these can then give hours of pleasure watching the birds and diaries or journals can be made recording their success and the birds seen. The food necessary to feed the birds can also be a source of activity as the tables will need to be checked for water and nuts and restocked as necessary and "fat balls" can be made out of bacon rind and left over fat to feed them (a less messy option is to string together cereal loops such as "Cheerios" to feed them or to stuff pine cones with peanut butter etc.).

In the last paragraph I mentioned making bird tables etc. but depending on the skill level and interest it also possible to make other things from wood and these kits are readily available. They range in difficulty from ornamental boxes and hanging mobiles to wooden toys, boats and planes and there is usually something that will suit all personalities and abilities.

Handicrafts also include making things in clay, plasticine and dough (one cup flour, half a cup of salt and a little water, modelling whatever shapes, objects and ornaments you desire and then slowly baking it on a low heat to harden it). Once the model has been made the next step is to paint or decorate it (and if you don't want to make something you can always decorate eggs!) which again improve the co-ordination of the hands and the eyes.

Needle craft covers a wide range of activities as well ranging from crocheting to knitting to sewing to cross point and so on – and it is not just a female activity as many of my male patients are also avid fans when it comes to a knitting needle!

Outdoor Activities

It is always nice to be outside for a change of scenery and even with our weather there is always something to do and they don't all have to be expensive. Starting with the cheapest activities first it is always nice to go for a walk exploring old buildings or churches, or just enjoying the countryside – bird watching, walking a dog, throwing a ball etc. or the sea side – walking on the beach, sitting in the sun, eating an ice cream or just spending time with family and friends. You can then do all the things that used to thrill you as a child that you haven't done for years and fly kites, make snowmen, collect shells etc. – none of which cost anything.

It is possible to visit libraries to look for books or CDs, get involved with shopping trips (often just being asked to participate or for an opinion makes everyone feel worthwhile). Take bus journeys through town to visit places from the past or historical bus tours are usually a good source of interest. You can visit aquariums, the zoo, museums, art galleries and even "pick you own" fruit and vegetables farms provide a day out (and you have something to show for it at the end!).

Cooking Activities

As a man, I have been told (and I find this hard to believe) there is always something to do in the kitchen!

Activities can include peeling vegetables or potatoes (especially the ones you have grown), shelling peas or beans, shelling nuts, preparing salads or fruit salads, decorating cakes, mixing the ingredients for cakes, bread etc., making jams, chutneys or sauces, pickling or preserving. The list is endless as long as there is a little supervision and the ingredients are placed to hand nearby, helping out in the kitchen can prove stimulating, productive and worthwhile.

Activities To Help Around The Home

There are many activities and chores that can be done around the home that will allow people to feel involved and wanted. There are for example always things that need sorting out whether these are old newspapers and magazines to be put in the recycling, washing jars and bottles to recycle, sorting out socks into pairs as they come out of the washing machine or sorting out playing cards, buttons, screws, nuts and bolts, folding clothes, writing name tags, signing letters or bills.

If that wasn't enough to get you thinking of your own ideas there is also cutting out adverts or coupons, winding up string, cotton onto reels, wool into balls, polishing things (usually it is better if they are not fragile, valuable or sentimental so things like large brass ornaments are ideal). The list goes on and on and it is really only limited by your own imagination!

In the early stages of dementia the use of memory joggers or prompters may be helpful so that things remain as normal as possible. There are many different ways in which you can improve both cognition and memory by the use of aids, but the best types to think about should not only be clear to use, easy to carry out or perform and actually help to jog the memory and /or minimise confusion.

I would recommend that you read through the following list of ideas and see which ones may be applicable to your unique circumstance.

Remember that every case is individual and that people experience memory difficulties in different ways and therefore not all of these tips may be appropriate to your situation.

Memory Joggers
- Ideas That May Help

1. The first thing to remember is that everyone has memory lapses (some more than others!), and at one time or another we have all gone into a room only to have forgotten why – and then to have remembered once again after we have left and gone elsewhere! The reason I mention this is this; as you will recall the more you got stressed at the time about trying to remember, the worse the situation became and the harder it was to recall what it was you were after. The same is true for those that you may be caring for. Therefore, avoid rushing or putting pressure on either yourself (in future!) or the family member or friend you may be caring for as this only makes the situation worse and makes remembering that much harder.

2. Focus on one activity at a time and keep to it until it is complete. To misquote an old proverb "a job completed by hand is worth two in the bush (or future!).

3. Buy a notebook, diary and pen for yourself, relative or friend to write down important information, conversations, shopping lists, things to do or instructions.

   This can also be kept by the telephone so that messages / conversations can be written down as they take place and important information will not be forgotten (also keep important telephone numbers by the 'phone so that they are always in easy reach.

4. Using your notebook (or a wipe clean blackboard or whiteboard) it is also useful to leave notes, messages and reminders behind (if you are a carer) when you are going out informing your loved one of where you are going, why you are going and when you will return.

5. Keep a visible watch or clock (with a large face for easy viewing) and calendar so that changes in the day, date, month and year can be noted and recorded. Use the calendar to make a note of all the important dates, anniversaries, appointments etc. which once recorded can then be used as a reminder. Cross out or mark off the days as they pass to keep a visual record of the time, date, seasons etc.

6. Make sure that you get a daily newspaper and then throw out the old ones. This will help you to keep track of the days and establish a routine whilst keeping your mind active – and you never know you may always find something of interest in it as well!

7. It is possible to get pill dispensers or holders for tablets that also have the days of the weeks and times on them – this is again another useful way to keep track of time but more importantly they can be vital in helping the sufferer keep track of taking the right pill at the right time.
It is also possible to either set an alarm clock / radio or purchase an electronic reminder to sound at the appropriate time for medications to be taken – again handy for establishing a daily routine.

8. There is nothing wrong with routine, doing things in the same order or by habit and using check-lists if necessary as this helps to keep up some independence and self reliance wherever possible.

9. Tidy up and remove any junk from cupboards, work surfaces and drawers (I believe they call this de-cluttering or being "minimalistic"!) as this helps to minimise confusion for those being cared for. Avoid re-organising familiar things as this may create confusion and try to keep keys, glasses, money, remote controls etc. in the same place as this helps establish a routine and a pattern of knowing where the most common objects are.

10. Label all drawers and cupboards so that the person you are caring for knows where important things are kept. Make sure that you keep each item in one place as this helps establish a routine. Don't hide things (also known as "putting things in a safe place") as it may cause confusion.

Before I leave the section on mental activity and improved thinking, I just want to say a little word about stress and depression. Studies have shown a clear link between depression and a decrease in memory recall. One important study has shown that the leading cause of deteriorating memory amongst their volunteers was depression and not in fact Alzheimer's disease.

Therefore it is all the more reason to keep both the sufferer and the carer as active both mentally and physically as possible to alleviate boredom and prevent depression from setting in. If you would like to try to improve depression with the use of supplements it is worth noting that vitamins B1, B3, B6, B12 and biotin are naturally involved in the production of serotonin – the good mood hormone!

One final word for the carers (and also the sufferer), I read in a research paper that when they are trying to find individuals for studies and trials who are suffering stress the first people they seek are those that are caring for someone with Alzheimer's – because they feel there isn't anything more stressful than being a carer in these circumstances.

Unfortunately, when the body is undergoing stress it produces tremendous amounts of the hormone cortisol which damages the part of the brain involved with memory production (the hippocampus). One of the research papers published in the Journal of Neuroscience in 2006 actually stated that high levels of cortisol caused Alzheimer's disease and were not present because of it as had been previously thought (**30**).

For this reason I would recommend that you consider taking up some of the many relaxation techniques that are on offer whether it is relaxation CDs, hypnotherapy, tai-chi or yoga. You will definitely feel the benefit both now and in the long run!

The Affects of Smoking and Alcohol Consumption On Alzheimer's Disease

The next couple of areas I want to cover are fairly controversial so I don't intend to dwell on them too much. Everyone has their own ideas about smoking and alcohol – should you / shouldn't you, how much is too much etc. and even the official guidelines seem to change on a weekly basis.

So, for the next couple of paragraphs I will give you my views and I will try to be impartial (as ever!).

Smoking and Alzheimer's Disease

What better way to start than with something that everyone has strong opinions about and with something that everyone knows their view is right. Views about cigarettes are like a "tinder-box" waiting to be ignited (excuse the pun) so I might as well have my say.

The good news with smoking is that the opinions on it with regards to Alzheimer's disease are mixed – so everyone has chance to be right!

Initially it was believed that smoking offered a form of protection against Alzheimer's but unfortunately this is now known to be only half true. The good news is that if you have one of the genetic types that makes you predisposed to Alzheimer's disease then smoking may offer some protection against the condition.

In those people that have the APOE epsilon 4 gene (a gene linked to the development of Alzheimer's disease) researchers found that smoking had no effect with regards to increasing the risk of developing Alzheimer's for people with this gene and that it may actually lower the incidence of Alzheimer's amongst these particular individuals **(31)**. Unfortunately if you do not have this gene then the risk of Alzheimer's disease is increased by almost 2½ times.

The reasons for this are unknown and further research is needed. It is known that smoking can cause a reduction in the blood supply throughout the body and as mentioned earlier strokes and heart disease are all causative factors in the onset of Alzheimer's disease and dementia. Smoking also causes oxidative stress (or cell aging) and hence further increases the risks.

On the positive side it was thought that smoking had an effect on the brain's neurotransmitters (the chemicals that make it work) preventing them from being broken down as quickly during the process of dementia or Alzheimer's disease. Studies have shown the positive benefits of nicotine (although the studies tend to use nicotine injections) protecting subjects from Alzheimer's as it is believed that nicotine improves the bodies responsiveness to acetylcholine – an important chemical needed for memory formation.

I could find only a couple of research papers that stated that smoking may actually be of benefit to Alzheimer's sufferers.

One of them in particular (and some of you may like this paper a lot) shows positive effects from smoking and no negative effects of alcohol consumption on dementia / Alzheimer's **(32)**.

Unfortunately, this tends to be a lone voice amongst the research papers so I would not put to much weight behind it – particularly when it tells you that the more you smoke and the longer you have smoked the better it is for you and one of the main researchers is named Graves!

This brings us nicely on to the effects of alcohol and this time I may have some better news for you!

Alcohol and Alzheimer's Disease

Many researchers have shown that excessive alcohol consumption (this is three or more drinks daily) can lead to a decline in cognition and alcohol related dementia – but the link between alcohol and Alzheimer's tends to be nothing but positive and moderate drinking has benefits for this condition and the other types of dementia as well. In fact, light-to-moderate alcohol consumption (one to three alcoholic drinks a day) was associated with a 42% risk reduction of all types dementia and a 70% reduction in risk of vascular dementia (dementia caused by a series of small strokes).

Researchers believe that alcohol consumption may have a direct effect on brain activity by stimulating the release of the chemical acetylcholine in the hippocampus area of the brain – the area of the brain involved with converting short term memories into long term memories – and the increase in acetylcholine release actual enhances the memory and learning processes. So, in this instance, it really is true that "a little of what you fancy does you good" however just remember that a high alcohol intake inhibits acetylcholine production and therefore reverses this process **(33)** – so don't over do it!

Now that I've allowed you a drink or two it is time to turn our attention to your diet for a quick look at a few dos and don'ts.

Section Three

Before I continue with the section on how supplements can be beneficial to Alzheimer's disease and dementia, I first want to look at how a few simple dietary changes can prove of tremendous value to improving your memory and preventing the onset of these conditions.

To start with I want to take a very broad look at your diet and just how much food you are eating and its possible consequences.

Any food that you eat is broken down to do two main things – provide nourishment and provide fuel. The nourishment is important as it is the material that repairs and regenerates your body hopefully keeping it working at an optimum. The fuel side of the equation is also vital as this provides you with the energy to function. There is no point being 100% healthy if you don't feel like doing anything and there is no point having the energy to do anything and everything you choose if your body and mind isn't up to it.

However, there is a drawback with the fuel side of things....

Anything that you eat is broken down during digestion and during this process free radicals are formed. These chemicals immediately start to damage all the cells of the body and it is these chemicals that are believed to be behind the ageing process. Therefore, the more food you eat the more free radicals you produce and, in effect, the more damage you are doing to yourself.

It was this idea that led researchers at the Columbia University in New York City to conduct a study **(1)** into the eating habits of almost 1000 people to see if there was any connection between a high calorie diet and the onset of dementia. At the start of the trial none of the volunteers showed any signs of dementia but at the end of it almost 25% of the group showed signs of Alzheimer's disease or dementia. Of those that did it was found that those that consumed the highest number of calories were almost one and a half times more likely to develop these conditions than those that were on a low fat / low calorie diet!

More calories equalled more dementia!

What was even more startling was that those of the subjects that carried the apolipoprotein-E gene variant known as apoE e-4 (which I mentioned earlier is one of the known risk factors to developing Alzheimer's) were twice as likely to develop the condition if they were on a high calorie diet. What is even more important is that approximately one in five people carry this gene!

This study supports another that showed obesity as a risk factor to developing Alzheimer's disease. Research published in the Journal of Alzheimer's Disease **(2)** showed that obesity can aggravate or contribute to the severity or progression of Alzheimer's as it is believed the fatter a person, the higher the levels of beta-amyloid (a sticky protein substance that can build up in the brain of Alzheimer's sufferers) are in their blood.

What is surprising is that further studies have shown that the main culprit with regards to diet is **the amount of carbohydrates that that are consumed**. Studies carried out on mice (with the mouse equivalent of Alzheimer's!) have shown that restricting carbohydrate intake specifically can halt or even reverse the symptoms of Alzheimer's disease. One study in particular which appeared in the July 2006 issue of the Journal of Biological Chemistry was the first to show that restricting carbohydrates may prevent Alzheimer's disease by triggering activity in the brain associated with a long life **(3)**.

We mentioned earlier about the effects of diabetes on dementia and Alzheimer's but you don't necessarily have to have diabetes to be at risk from the effects of uncontrolled blood sugar. The brain is the largest consumer of energy in your body and almost one quarter of the fuel you make goes to "feed" it. Eating refined carbohydrates, also known as "white poison" as they are white sugar and white flour (in other words bread, pasta biscuits etc.) causes your blood sugar to fluctuate widely and effects the functioning of your brain (and in particularly memory) as it cannot receive the nutrients it needs to perform properly. Too few nutrients can lead to nerve damage and in extreme cases nerve death.

To counteract this the body produces chemicals to try to stabilise the blood sugar and it does this by producing a hormone called cortisol (which I mentioned earlier when I talked about stress). Cortisol further destroys nerve cells and brain tissue – especially in the hippocampus part of the brain which is important for memory storage.

Now, before you start panicking about having to stop eating carbohydrates altogether and follow the Atkins diet or something similar I will show you some very simple ways to reduce your carbohydrates and further improve your health at the same time.

The easiest way to reduce your carbohydrate intake is to stop drinking fizzy drinks, flavoured water, energy drinks and fruit juice drinks (that way you reduce your intake of high fructose corn syrup, glucose and fructose) and to use sparingly sugar and honey (honey is a medicine not a food!).

A study reported from the American Society for Biochemistry and Molecular Biology **(4)** suggests that drinks with high sugar content have been linked to the increase in risk of Alzheimer's. The study found that mice that were fed a 10% sugar solution (or the equivalent of about 5 cans of fizzy drink) showed a decline in learning and memory retention, and their brains contained over twice as many amyloid plaque deposits – a hallmark of Alzheimer's.

As I have already mentioned, Alzheimer's has already been strongly linked to obesity and the authors of this research paper were unsure as to whether the sugar solution itself caused the memory deficits and the onset of Alzheimer's, or if it was the result of the increased calories and increased weight brought on by the sugar water.

So, the question is – what can you drink instead? Well, to help you out here are three suggestions that can make a positive difference to your mental well being.

Green tea has a unique antioxidant called EGCG that is able to convert the amyloid plaques associated with Alzheimer's disease into a less damaging molecule. By converting these plaques in such a way it is believed that green tea should help slow down (if not help prevent) the progression of the disease. Green tea has a far higher concentration of these important antioxidants and to have a therapeutic effect you would need to only drink four cups a day. However, if you prefer you can also drink normal **black tea** (which contains about a fifth of the antioxidant concentration) but you would need to drink much, much more – and you will be unable to add milk as this has been shown to destroy this valuable compound.

Researchers have found that **Rooibos tea** protects the nervous system and the brain especially against the damage from free radicals **(5)**. Rooibos (as well as **Oolong tea**) contain flavonoids and polyphenols both of which are powerful antioxidants and free radical scavengers (which can lead to dementia and degenerative conditions such as Alzheimer's disease) as they can prevent the breakdown of proteins and cell mutation.

Unfortunately, much of this activity is lost in the processing of the tea and what is left is not very water soluble – in effect making Rooibos half as powerful an antioxidant as black tea (which as you will recall is even less powerful than green tea!)

If tea isn't your cup of tea (no pun intended) then you will be pleased to know the benefits have also been seen in coffee drinkers. In fact, two very good articles show that coffee and caffeine consumption have a great response in reducing the risk of dementia and Alzheimer's disease in particular. A study published in the European Journal of Clinical Nutrition **(6)** suggests that coffee drinkers may be protected from mild memory and thinking problems that come with old age, whilst a 2002 **(7)** found that people who consumed more caffeine in middle age appeared to be protected from developing Alzheimer's later on.

It is believed (from work done on mice) that the caffeine may reduce the levels of plaque that forms in the brains of Alzheimer's sufferers as caffeine can stop bad cholesterol moving from the blood stream into the brain. Although it is speculation as to the effects in humans researchers cannot see any reason why the effects and therefore the results shouldn't be the same.

Regardless of whether coffee plays a role in the prevention of Alzheimer's or not other benefits from drinking coffee have been noted. These include a reduced risk of type 2 diabetes, Parkinson's disease, cirrhosis and cancer of the liver and even suicide! Therefore with all these benefits it may be worth drinking a cup or two anyway!

Dr. Robert Krikorian, a researcher from the University of Cincinnati College of Medicine, has said that drinking **Concord grape juice** shows a positive benefit in slowing cognitive decline (his very words were "a simple, easy-to-incorporate dietary intervention that could improve or protect memory function, such as drinking Concord grape juice daily, may be beneficial for the ageing population"). He believes that it is the high polyphenol (anti-oxidant) content found in the skin of the grapes which lowers the risk of developing Alzheimer's disease.

His research has shown that after only 12 weeks of drinking 15 to 21 ounces of Concord grape juice, participants in his study showed a "significant improvement" in learning ability and that those who've had issues with short-term memory loss would benefit in making grape juice an every day part of their diet.

If you are unable to find Concord grape juice then other research has shown that **any fruit or vegetable juice** is beneficial in reducing your risk of Alzheimer's. A study published in the American Journal of Medicine **(8)** showed that drinking 3 glasses of fruit and / or vegetable juice could reduce the risk of developing Alzheimer's or dementia by 75%. Although the study did not specify which juices were consumed it did rule out other lifestyle factors – leaving only the juice as the preventative factor.

The reason for this preventative action is believed to be due to the high concentration of antioxidants (or polyphenols and flavonoids to be technical) found in the juices that have come from the skins of the fruit or vegetables. As well as the benefits in cognition, fruit and vegetable juices have also been found to reduce the effects of ageing and have anti-cancer properties as well – so more reason to tuck in!

Whilst we are discussing the role of a low carbohydrate diet I must mention a few words about dietary fat. If you are reducing the amount of carbohydrates that you eat, then very often your consumption of protein and fat increases along with the resultant worry about cholesterol.

I must make it clear from the start that as a practitioner of complementary health techniques I am not in favour of "statin" drugs to reduce cholesterol and I am especially concerned about their use in the treatment of Alzheimer's disease and dementia as the results are extremely mixed.

A study published in the Journals of Gerontology **(9)** showed that the use of statins is associated with a lower prevalence of dementia and has a positive impact on the progression of cognitive impairment. Whilst another study in The Lancet **(10)** showed that patients given statin medication whether or not they had high cholesterol had a substantially lowered risk of developing dementia.

However, other studies have shown that there is no improvement in dementia when taking statins or a reduced risk of developing the condition and other studies have shown that certain statin medications can actually make dementia conditions worse **(11, 12)** and have even shown that a low good cholesterol level is a risk factor for developing dementia and memory deterioration **(13)**.

Unfortunately, an estimated 1 in 8-10 people on statin medication will experience side effects that include muscle pain, memory lapses, depression, mood swings, sexual dysfunction, damage to the liver and kidneys and strokes. So much so that one leading doctor has warned that patients should be told that "the reduced cardiovascular risk will be replaced by other serious illnesses".

With that it mind I wonder if any perceived benefits are actually worth it.

I would like to stress that a diet high in saturated fats and trans fats i.e. chips, crisps, burgers, biscuits, cakes, ice cream, pastry and anything deep-fried may result in these fats being absorbed into your cell membranes and into your red blood cells. This results in reduced blood flow and a hardening of the artery walls thereby decreasing the circulation to the vital organs of the body (and it is my belief that they are all vital otherwise you wouldn't have them!). This reduces the amount of oxygen and other nutrients that may get to your brain, for example, seriously affecting the way that it works.

One way to counteract this is to increase the amount of polyunsaturated oils that you consume which have been shown to increase red blood cell flexibility and activity and improve the mental functioning of those patients with Alzheimer's.

My recommendation is that you should avoid trans fats and saturated fats as much as possible (as these have been shown to increase the risk of Alzheimer's disease especially amongst those with a genetic predisposition to the condition) and use olive oil where ever possible. The "Mediterranean" style diet as it is known has been shown to be of benefit in reducing the risk of Alzheimer's and dementia in general.

Recommendation

The Mediterranean diet is abundant in virgin olive oil, high quantities of fruit, vegetables, nuts and seeds, fish and wholegrain pulses and cereals.

The only drawback to this type of diet is for those people that may suffer from a gluten sensitivity (gluten is found in most cereals especially wheat, barley, oats and rye). A recent study in the journal Neurology (14) that early-stage dementia may be linked with sensitivity to gluten and that these symptoms improved in nine out of the ten patients when they were given a gluten-free diet.

Having briefly touched on the Mediterranean diet, it is worth saying a little bit about various oils and how they can be used to improve your memory and reduce your risk of dementia – especially the essential fatty acids as they are vital to good health.

Numerous studies have shown that people with a low level of omega-3 fatty acids (docosahexaenoic acid or DHA to be precise) are at a greater risk of developing dementia than those that have higher levels of this fatty acid. Not only that, but the higher your levels of this fatty acid the lower your risk of developing the condition. It also works both ways – too little increases the risk, the greater the levels the lower the risk (and by as much as 50 percent!).

This fatty acid is easily obtained both naturally in the diet from cold water fish such as mackerel, tuna, salmon and herring as well as seeds and nuts (in particular flax seeds and walnuts) and through supplementation. It is well worth adding to your diet as it has shown numerous health benefits – not all of which are to do with memory. Apart from helping to create brain tissue (helping with memory and learning), reduce the build up of Alzheimer's plaques **(15)** and allowing the nervous system to work properly by supporting how nerves fire, it also improves vision, removes inflammation and helps control allergies.

Omega 6 fatty acids derived from seeds such as hemp, pumpkin, sunflower and sesame and wheat germ oil have also been shown to reduce heart problems, lower cholesterol and improve long term memory **(16)**.

Finally in this section I must refer you to a web page that talks about the hidden danger of artificial sweeteners – www.health-n-energy.com/ARTICLES/9artsweet.htm.

This article is too long to write in its entirety but below is a brief extract that you may find of interest which talks about the effects of these sweeteners and in particular Aspartame:

"Dr. Russell Blaylock, neurosurgeon and author of the book "Excitotoxins: The Taste That Kills" states that "The ingredients stimulates the neurons of the brain to death, causing brain damage of varying degrees."

Dr. H.J. Roberts, diabetic specialist and world expert on aspartame poisoning, has also written a book entitled "Defense Against Alzheimer's Disease". Dr. Roberts tells how aspartame poisoning is escalating Alzheimer's Disease, and indeed it is...

According to the Conference of the American College of Physicians, "We are talking about a plague of neurological diseases caused by this deadly poison". Dr. Roberts realized what was happening when aspartame was first marketed. He said his "diabetic patients presented memory loss, confusion, and severe vision loss". At the conference doctors admitted that they did not know why. They had wondered why seizures were rampant (the phenylalanine in aspartame breaks down the seizure threshold and depletes serotonin, which causes **manic depression, panic attacks, rage and violence**)."

I leave it up to you discretion whether or not you continue to use sweeteners but I try to get all of my patients of off them at every opportunity.

Section Four

As I discussed earlier, improving your lifestyle, partaking in a little physical and mental exercise, keeping a check on your overall health and improving your diet will dramatically lessen your chances of developing (as well as slowing the rate of progression) of Alzheimer's and the other dementias. But sometimes that isn't enough and a couple of little further steps will pay you big dividends.

In this next part we are going to look at how taking vitamin and herbal supplements will improve your cognition and reduce your chances of developing Alzheimer's disease and other dementias (and improve them if you are already suffering) beyond belief!

Vital Vitamins for Protecting yourself from Alzheimer's Disease and Dementia.

The Vitamin C and E Combination

An article published in the International Journal of Geriatric Psychiatry **(1)** showed that all Alzheimer's sufferers had low blood plasma concentrations of vitamin C no matter how good their diet was. It also showed and that the lower the concentrations the worse their thinking or cognition was but they were unable to explain why this was. It maybe due to problems with absorption, or the vitamin C is being used up more quickly amongst those suffering with dementia but regardless of the reason they knew it was important.

This study supports the theory that vitamin C is vital in reducing the damage done by free radicals within the body and the brain itself. Vitamin C is a powerful anti-oxidant and coupled with vitamin E the results are even far more impressive (but I will cover that in just a moment)..

Researchers have also discovered that vitamin C enhances the effect of medications used to treat dementia allowing the drugs to pass more easily into the brain and therefore have a greater effect. A study published in the Journal of Medicinal Chemistry in 2002 showed that certain drugs were prevented from entering the brain by the blood-brain barrier (a control filter that prevents harmful materials entering the brain and central nervous system) but with the addition of vitamin C this filtering mechanism was overcome.

As well as being a powerful anti-oxidant and removing free radicals from the body, vitamin C is also involved in over 300 hundred metabolic processes that are vital for health. Some of these processes are extremely important in the prevention of dementia and Alzheimer's. For example, vitamin C lowers your level of bad cholesterol whilst raising your level of good cholesterol, helps your body detox heavy metals, helps in the metabolisms of carbohydrates, lowers blood pressure and reduces atherosclerosis or hardening of the arteries.

So, regardless of how good your diet is a supplementation of vitamin C may prove very beneficial. If you are going to try a supplement you may as well add vitamin E to – you'll be glad that you did (as I will show you now)...

A study in the American Journal of Clinical Nutrition **(2)** showed that vitamin E intake was inversely proportional to the incidence of Alzheimer's disease – i.e. the more you took the less likely you were to suffer from the condition. The study also showed that increased levels of vitamin E could reverse the symptoms of Alzheimer's.

Vitamin E also acts as a powerful antioxidant by neutralizing free radicals in the body that cause tissue and cell damage. As well as this vitamin E also contributes to a healthy circulatory system and aids in proper blood clotting and may decrease the risk of Coronary Artery Disease (CAD) by slowing the development of atherosclerosis.

It therefore makes sense to take a supplement of vitamins C and E – but it makes even more sense to take them together! In fact, a study in 2006 by the Johns Hopkins University showed that those who took a combination of vitamin C and E supplements over a six-year period had a significantly lower risk of developing Alzheimer's.

Recommendation

A daily dose of 2500-3000mg of vitamin C and up to 800mg of vitamin E may prove beneficial in reducing and slowing the effects of Alzheimer's and other dementias.

Ibuprufen and Vitamins C and E

Before I leave the subject of vitamins C and E, I want to discuss a number of trials that have mentioned adding ibuprofen to this combination. Researchers from the John Hopkins University shared their findings at a recent meeting of the American Academy of Neurology and they reported that adding ibuprofen to the vitamin C and E mix resulted in the subjects showing no mental decline over 8 years. All groups improved but those with a high risk of developing Alzheimer's disease showed greatest improvement.

It is believed that the vitamins act as anti-inflammatory agents and therefore protect the brain whilst the ibuprofen destroys clumps of plaque that have already developed in the brain. The researchers added that "if patients seem to be at high risk, such as having several family members with Alzheimer's disease or with early memory loss, they are likely to benefit the most from the triple-combination therapy."

There is nothing new in this study as similar studies by Johns Hopkins University and the National Institute on Ageing published in the Journal of Neurology in 1997 showed that the risk of developing Alzheimer's disease can be reduced by as much as 60 percent by frequent consumption of ibuprofen over two years or longer and that even shorter use could reduce the risk by as much as 35 percent **(3)**.

There are some drawbacks to this "good" news...

Firstly, no improvement was made in those subjects taking aspirin which is a more powerful anti-inflammatory than ibuprofen. Therefore the mechanisms behind ibuprofen's actions are not yet fully understood. The Alzheimer's Disease Anti-inflammatory Prevention Trial (ADAPT) in 2007 **(4)** tested the daily use of two non steroidal anti-inflammatory (NSAID) pain killers – Naproxen and Celebrex on over 2,000 elderly subjects each with a family history of Alzheimer's and they found no benefit at all. In fact, the subjects in the Naproxen group actually scored lower on cognitive function tests than subjects in the placebo group and also (more importantly) the study had to be stopped after 3 years when other studies found that Celebrex increased the risk of heart attack.

Secondly, I am always wary when researchers find new combinations of drugs or vitamins or whatever that do wonderful things and then they want to start marketing or selling their own!

Thirdly, and I believe most importantly, ibuprofen can cause peptic ulcers and kidney damage. It would not be a good idea to develop these two conditions whilst trying to protect yourself from something you may not get – unless, of course, you are already taking ibuprofen for another reason in which case you may enjoy an anti-Alzheimer's effect as a bonus.

Recommendation

If you decide to try Ibuprofen for its protective role in Alzheimer's disease then firstly consult your medical practitioner and secondly restrict your dosage to no more than 100mg of ibuprofen a day.

The Benefits of B Vitamins

All the B vitamins play a role in improving and maintaining brain health and even a mild deficiency may lead to memory loss, confusion, anxiety, depression and sleep disorders. I regularly recommend that my patients take either a vitamin B complex or the B vitamins individually and the research is there to back the benefits of this. In 2005 the United States Department of Agriculture monitored blood samples and cognitive function in more than 300 subjects for three years. They found that low levels of the B vitamins and high homocysteine concentrations were not only some of the best predictors of cognitive decline but are also extremely common in Alzheimer's patients.

Because of the importance of the B vitamins we are going to look at them individually starting with Folic acid.

Fun and Frolics with Folic Acid

Taking Folic acid (vitamin B9) may help ward off Alzheimer's disease by lowering the levels homocysteine found in the blood. Homocysteine is an amino acid found in meats that causes blood cells to clump together and cling to arterial walls. Too much homocysteine in the system can damage arterial walls and contribute to the development of atherosclerosis, a condition that may lead to an early heart attack.

One study in particular **(5)** showed that out of a group of 900 participants those with the highest levels of homocysteine at the start of the study were nearly twice as likely to develop dementia when they were re-assessed 8 years later. Not only has research shown the association between high homocysteine levels and the risk of dementia and Alzheimer's but they also found that homocysteine levels can be reduced by supplementing with Folic acid – so what better reason than to start taking some today?

Recommendation

I would recommend a daily dose of 400mcg of Folic acid as a maintenance dose and increasing this dose to 2,000mcg if you are showing signs of early dementia or have a family history of dementia.

Vitamin B 12 – The Vital B

Vitamin B12, also known as Cobalamin, works with Folic acid to produce healthy red blood cells and reduce homocysteine. Vitamin B12 also helps keeps your

central nervous system (i.e. all of your nerves) healthy –
as it has been shown to create, regenerate and sustain
nerve tissue.

Researchers have found that Alzheimer's patients
are often deficient in vitamin B12. This vitamin is vital in
protecting the brain against dementia and ageing by not
only reversing the nerve damage that are associated with
both conditions but by also regulating the action of other
chemical messengers, or neurotransmitters, in the brain
(6). Because of both these actions patients suffering with
Alzheimer's disease experienced improvements in
memory, emotions and their ability to communicate when
supplemented with vitamin B12.

Unfortunately, our bodies are only able to convert
1-2 % of the vitamin B12 we receive through our diets
(the only natural sources of vitamin B12 are animal
products) or supplementation into a form that our bodies
can use – a form called methylcobalamin. The good news
is that there is a now a form of methylcobalamin that
dissolves under your tongue and is rapidly absorbed into
the blood stream for direct use by the brain.

Recommendation

A recommended daily dose of between 1.5 – 2.5mg
of vitamin B12 sublingually (under the tongue)
may prove beneficial in the treatment of
Alzheimer's disease and other dementias.

Vitamin B12 works closely with Folic acid (vitamin B9) and Pyridoxine (vitamin B6) to convert food into energy. It also works with these B vitamins to protect your heart by removing homocysteine from the blood which if left to build up in large quantities is extremely detrimental to overall health.

Vitamin B6 – Pyridoxine.

Vitamin B6, also known as Pyroxidine, is used by numerous systems in the body including the brain, the nervous system, the gastrointestinal tract, the immune system and hormonal activity. It fact, vitamin B6 is believed to involved in more biological pathways than any other nutrient.

Vitamin B6, also plays a role in helping the body convert protein, fats and carbohydrates into energy. Together with Folic acid and B12 to reduce levels of homocysteine in the blood (helping to prevent atherosclerosis and lower the incidence of heart disease) whilst keeping red blood cells from forming potentially dangerous blood clots.

Vitamin B6 is also needed for the manufacture of certain neurotransmitters (such as serotonin and dopamine) which are required for normal nerve cell communication and it is because of this that B6 shows promising results with Alzheimer's disease, dementia and other neurological conditions such as seizures, chronic pain, depression, headache, and Parkinson's disease, ADD and mood swings **(7)**.

Researchers in Spain have shown that vitamin B6 deficiencies are associated with certain diseases that affect the elderly in particular: impaired cognitive function, Alzheimer's disease, cardiovascular disease and certain cancers **(8)**. Some of these problems may be related to the elevated homocysteine concentrations associated to vitamin B6 deficiency which we covered earlier, but there is also evidence for other yet unknown mechanisms by which a deficiency of vitamin B6 could increase the risk of these chronic diseases.

I recommend all my patients take a minimum of 100mg of vitamin B6 a day and these levels are further increased depending on history of mental illness, history of cancer or heart disease – and I suggest that this is a good place for you to start as well.

Recommendation

Vitamin B6 may cause side-effects including numbness of the hands and feet if taken in excessive doses (greater than 2,000mg daily)

However, dosages of up to 300mg may prove beneficial in the treatment of Alzheimer's disease and other neurological conditions.

Vitamin B6 reduces the effectiveness of Dilantin, a drug used to control epileptic seizures and therefore epileptics should avoid using this supplement.

Vitamin B3 – Niacin.

Niacin (or vitamin B3) comes in two forms nicotinic acid and niacinamide both of which have potential health benefits but it is normally the niacinamide form which is found in supplements – and it is that form and its benefits that I am going to discuss now.

Niacinamide not only helps prevent the development of insulin-dependent diabetes (which was one of the aggravating factors in cognitive decline and dementia we discussed earlier), but it may directly reduce the risk of Alzheimer's disease and age-related cognitive decline, according to a study published in the Journal of Neurology, Neurosurgery and Psychiatry **(9)**.

It is already known that a severe niacin deficiency can cause dementia through an illness caused pellagra, but this study aimed at testing whether high doses of niacin (either from food or supplementation) not only prevented dementia but reversed it.

What the researchers found was that a high intake of total niacin intake seemed to protect against both Alzheimer's and cognitive decline – and was linked to an 80% reduction in risk from both illnesses!

Inositol

Inositol was originally classified as a B vitamin (vitamin B8) until it was discovered that it could be manufactured by the body and "de-listed". Recent studies have shown that it is beneficial for most types of dementia, including Alzheimer's disease, as it is found in healthy brain tissue but in decreasing amounts in those patients suffering from cognitive decline. Inositol plays an important role in brain cell communication and function, the regulation of brain chemicals (the neurotransmitters serotonin and acetylcholine are both regulated by inositol and both are important for mood control and memory formation) and the prevention of atherosclerosis.

Several trials have shown that dosages of 10-12 grams daily even over a short period of time can lead to significant improvements in both language formation and retention as well as spacial orientation **(10)**. Other studies suggest that inositol may even have therapeutic effects in a wide spectrum of mental illnesses including depression, panic attacks and obsessive compulsive disorder **(11)**.

Recommendation

There is no recommended daily allowance for Inositol but in the therapeutic trials, dosages of up to 18 grams have been used without side-effects.

I would recommend a dosage of 12grams divided into 6 equal doses as being beneficial.

Come on Choline

Choline (considered to be part of the B vitamin complex) is the active ingredient in Lecithin and was first discovered in 1862 – but it was only in the last 20 years or so that it has been given any serious attention and its role in health really studied.

This ongoing work has shown that it is used by the body to manufacture and maintain healthy cell membranes and promote the manufacture of a specific neurotransmitter (brain chemical) that is used in memory storage.

This neurotransmitter is acetylcholine and a decrease in the amount of this chemical (as you will already know!) has been linked in numerous studies to Alzheimer's disease. It is believed that this deficit is due to a decrease of an enzyme that converts dietary choline in to acetylcholine in the brain and therefore would seem the ideal solution...

A study comparing the treatment of Alzheimer's patients with choline to a placebo group (that didn't receive choline) showed that after 6 months the control group improved whilst the placebo group worsened when their cognition was tested.

However, there is only one drawback with the use of choline.

Another study published in Methods and Findings in Experimental and Clinical Pharmacology (12) detected significant improvement in mental performance after only one month of treatment with CDP-choline (which is excellent) **but** only in subjects with early-onset Alzheimer's.

As with all supplements you intend to start, it is worth checking with you G.P. or healthcare practitioner before you do to ask their advice on dosage, but in studies using choline dosages of 1000mg and 400mg three times daily were used without problem. I would recommend a daily dose of up to 850mg which has been shown to be well tolerated but also necessary to prevent organ damage in many individuals

Beta-Carotene, the Carotenoids and Cognition.

Last but by no means least I want to turn our attention to the carotenoids.

The term carotene is used for several related substances which are responsible for the orange colour of carrots and many other fruits and vegetables (it also provides the yellow colour as well). Although not a vitamin as such, beta-carotene is regarded as a pro-vitamin as it can be converted by the digestive system into retinal, a form of vitamin A and it can also be stored in the liver and converted to vitamin A as needed. Even without conversion beta-carotene and the carotenoids are powerful anti-oxidants (removing free radicals from our bodies) and provide many health benefits in their own rights.

Even on a genetic level...

As I mentioned earlier when covering the causative factors of Alzheimer's, certain people have a genetic predisposition to developing Alzheimer's and they are the ones with the apolipoprotein E4 (ApoE4) gene. However, researchers have discovered that by increasing their daily intake of beta-carotene they can greatly reduce their risks.

Researchers from the UCLA School of Medicine recently studied a group of people with and without the ApoE4 gene for a period of 7 years and their results regarding beta-carotene were quite startling. What they found was that those that were genetically predisposed to Alzheimer's butt had the highest levels of beta-carotene had an 89 percent less risk of cognitive decline. Even those that didn't have this genetic predisposition had a reduced risk as well **(13)**.

Further studies have also shown that the longer the supplementation continues the greater the effects it has on improving cognition. **(14)**.

Beta-carotenes also play a role in decreasing cardiovascular disease. This is important not only because of the reduced risk of heart disease and strokes but because of the associated reduction in the risk of vascular dementia.

And there is even more good news.

The carotenoid group is made up of a number of different compounds and I will mention a few of them here as they are not only helpful but they are quite interesting in what they do...

Alpha-carotene – helps maintain healthy skin, bones, the immune system and good vision. It is also a powerful antioxidant and may help prevent cancer by stimulating cell-to-cell communication (a process which researchers now believe is necessary to ensure proper cell division).

Lutein – helps prevent macular degeneration (a condition usually affecting older people which results in a loss of vision in the centre of the field of vision because of damage to the retina.).

Lycopene – helps to prevent prostate, breast and pancreatic cancer and it also helps prevent heart disease. Low levels are associated with poor mental function **(15)**.

Zeaxanthin – helps prevent macular degeneration. Low levels are associated with poor mental function **(15)**.

Recommendation

Unlike vitamin A, there are no recorded levels at which the carotenoids may become toxic.

Researchers have found that 50mg of beta-carotene given on alternate days proved beneficial.

If that wasn't enough to get you thinking about a few supplements that may be beneficial to you – now we move on to the herbs!

<u>Curries Curative Powers</u>

Believe it or not, the humble curry is not only a very potent meal but also a very potent medicine!

Many curry dishes get their distinctive hot, spicy flavour and colour from curcumin – the yellow pigment derived from the turmeric root (a member of the ginger family). This herb has been used for thousands of years by practitioners of Ayurvedic medicine in India and the Far East for the treatment of indigestion, arthritis and kidney infections because it is a natural antioxidant and anti-inflammatory.

Following the revelation that India has one of the lowest rates of Alzheimer's in the world (with only 25 % of the number of sufferers as in the USA for example) attention is shifting towards curcumin benefits in treating Alzheimer's and other dementias. Although more research is needed before it can be categorically stated that curcumin prevents Alzheimer's (as the mechanism is still unclear) the research is heading in the direction that supports the rationale for the use of curcumin in clinical trials to prevent or treat Alzheimer's disease.

Research has shown that curcumin, even in low doses, suppresses oxidative damage, inflammation, cognitive deficits and amyloid accumulation by breaking up and untangling amyloid plaques in the brain. Because curcumin can cross the blood brain barrier (16) and bind to these plaques it also helps to prevent further plaque formation (17).

So should you rush out and start eating curry?

Well the answer to that is yes and no!

So with that in mind, I'll start with the negative press first of all and get that out of the way…

Although curcumin is used to treat stomach problems larger doses of it have been shown to cause and aggravate ulcers. It also causes the liver to release bile (which is ideal if you want to lower your cholesterol) but if you have any obstruction to the bile duct this may create problems. Also curcumin has blood thinning properties so it should be used with extreme caution by those taking anticoagulants or anti-inflammatory drugs.

On the plus side a study from the National University of Singapore showed that those who ate curry regularly generally scored higher on cognitive tests (having up to a 50% reduced risk of cognitive impairment) than those who ate it infrequently or never (18).

For those of you that may find it difficult to increase you curry intake (or wish to keep your friends), curcumin supplements are easily found over the Internet and in many health food stores and a daily dosage of 800-1000mg is recommended

---

Recommendation

Curcumin may aggravate certain stomach and bile duct conditions.

Caution is advised if taking anticoagulant or anti-inflammatory drugs

A curcumin supplement of up to 1000mg a day can be beneficial.

There are several other herbs that can be used either on their own or in combination to treat Alzheimer's (when they are combined their properties are further enhanced as I will cover later) and these are Ginkgo Biloba, Sage and Lemon Balm.

So let's move on – we have lots to cover...

Ginkgo Biloba and the Brain

Ginkgo Biloba is one of the oldest medical treatments known to man being derived from the leaves of the ginkgo (or Maidenhair) tree allegedly one of the oldest surviving plants on earth. It has been used successfully for thousands of years to treat various complaints and that was before science started to review it!

In early studies Ginkgo Biloba received a lot of bad press about not being effective in most of the things it had been previously used for (from increasing blood flow to restoring cognitive powers) – but many of those studies were faulty in that the sample sizes were too small, the trials didn't run for long enough and the dosages given to the subjects were too small.

But now all that is behind us…

In 2002, the Alzheimer's Society and the Cochrane Collaboration **(19)** published what was at the time the largest review on Ginkgo Biloba and dementia and it concluded that overall the studies showed convincing evidence that Ginkgo Biloba may benefit cognition,

115

emotional control and function, and A.D.L.s (or activities of daily living) in patients in the early stages of Alzheimer's.

More importantly, the review showed that often these benefits occurred on dosages of less than 200mg a day and in under 3 months. And as an added bonus no adverse reactions (or side-effects) were noted!

In practice it has long been recognised that Ginkgo Biloba does have a positive effect not only on increasing cognition and memory in Alzheimer's and other dementias (by thinning the blood, dilating blood vessels and protecting nerves from further deterioration) due to it's anti-oxidant properties but also in reducing some of the other symptoms (such as emotional volatility) associated with these various conditions **(20)**.

One of the reasons for it ability to help control emotional instability is that it has a potent effect on the regulation of neurotransmitters (the chemicals in the brain that help to regulate how both it and the body functions). Dr Pierre Le Bars from the New York Institute for Medical Research has reported exciting research on its place in the management of Alzheimer's and other dementias, which he believes are linked to improved cell communication.

The importance of this work has led to an article in the *Quarterly Review of Natural Medicine* that Ginkgo is "one of the clinician's most useful tools for slowing cognitive decline in the elderly."

And it gets even better!

Additional research (from the Human Cognitive Neuroscience Unit at Northumbria University) has shown that the effects of Ginkgo Biloba are enhanced further with the addition of Ginseng along side it. The two researchers involved with this additional study found that when these two herbs were given in a combined dose concentration improved within the hour (there is further information on how these two herbs act together in the next few pages).

One word of caution though. Because Ginkgo has such strong (positive) effects on circulation care must be taken if on aspirin or other medications to thin the blood. Usually dosages of up to 200mg a day are safe but consult your G.P. before starting to use Ginkgo Biloba as a supplement.

Recommendation

Caution is advised if taking aspirin or other medications to thin the blood.

A Ginkgo Biloba supplement of up to 200mg a day can be beneficial.

Red Ginseng

Red ginseng (also called panax or Asian ginseng) is a powerful adaptogen which means it helps the body cope with stress and increase endurance. It is also capable of improving cognitive function and enhancing memory. As well as this, two of ginseng's chemical components have also shown promising results in regenerating brain cells and pathways in laboratory experiments. This is highly significant because these brain cells are typically destroyed by Alzheimer's disease **(21)**.

Another important role that red ginseng plays in memory and cognitive improvement is its ability to increase the amount of acetycholine that is formed in the brain **(22)** which is one of the more important neurotransmitters or brain chemicals associated with memory and learning.

Although ginseng is not recommended for patients suffering from high blood pressure for everyone else a daily supplementation of 200 – 400 mg of ginseng extract is well tolerated.

Recommendation

A daily supplement of 400mg of ginseng extract may improve cognition and memory in those suffering from Alzheimer's disease and other dementias.

Ginseng is not recommended for those suffering from high blood pressure.

Further gains can be made when ginseng is taken together with Ginkgo Biloba with improvements often being seen within the hour. This is because combined together Ginkgo Biloba improves the power of concentration, while ginseng sharpens the memory.

Dr Scholey a researcher from Human Cognitive Neuroscience Unit at Northumbria University said that scientists have for a long time been looking for a drug that improves both memory and concentration as "normally when you speed people up you lose a bit of accuracy, or if they are more accurate they take longer to respond" and with these two herbs combined he believes they may have found one. He has commented that "these two herbs added together synergistically in a remarkable way" meaning that the combined effects were far greater than the effects of both the individual herbs added together!

In his research, participants took a 960mg combination of both ginseng and Ginkgo Biloba (approximately 580mg of ginseng and 380mg Ginkgo Biloba) or a 60% - 40% mix.

Another study from China again showed the combined effects of ginseng and Ginkgo Biloba on enhancing the production of acetylcholine in the brains of laboratory animals that had been injected with amyloid plaques. In this study, the animals were given the ginseng and ginkgo extracts daily for a month and at the end of the study the extracts significantly increased the amount of acetylcholine in the animal's brains, allowing for good cognitive function.

These results have also been replicated in human studies where an extract of only ginseng administered over a 12 week period showed dramatic results in cognition improvement in those suffering from Alzheimer's **(23)**.

<u>"Sage" Isn't A Name Given To The Wise For No Reason!</u>

Sage has been recognised of use as a treatment for cognitive decline since the middle of the 17th century yet it is only now being looked at as a treatment for modern day dementias.

In 2003 it was shown to improve memory, orientation and learning **(24)** in patients with mild to moderate Alzheimer's disease. It also has an effect in decreasing the agitation and anxiety that sufferers often present with (especially when it is coupled with lemon balm) **(25)**. Like many of the other treatments we have discussed, sage boosts the amount of acetylcholine in the brain (which is very often depleted in Alzheimer's disease) by blocking the enzyme AchE (acetylcholinesterase) that breaks it down.

There are very few contra-indications in the use of sage for the treatment foe Alzheimer's and for that reason I would certainly start adding it to your cooking. I would also suggest that sage tincture be taken (in water) at a dose of about 20 drops three times per day.

Lemon Balm For The Not So "Barmy"

Lemon Balm is another useful herb to not only control memory decline and mood fluctuations but also slow their progression. It does this by controlling free radical damage as well as maintaining levels of acetylcholine which promotes memory and helps transmit messages between brain cells.

Remarkably, lemon balm is one of the most power memory herbs and is actually able to regenerate brain cells as well as making them more receptive to acetylcholine which starts to decline in quantity both with Alzheimer's and age.

Researchers in Iran showed that after a four month use of lemon balm subjects demonstrated a significant improvement in their symptoms – including memory and cognitive abilities – compared to a group that received a placebo **(26)**.

The recommended daily dose of lemon balm can vary anywhere up to 1000mg because lower dosages promote calmness and mood control and higher levels may sometimes cause a decrease in alertness (but an initial starting dose of around 450mg is not uncommon).

For this reason, it is necessary to speak to your health provider about a maintenance dose that is suitable for you as you will need to monitor the effect that it is has on both mood control and mental alertness **(27)**.

Recommendation

A Lemon Balm supplement of up to 1000mg a day can be beneficial.

Caution needs to be taken with larger doses as it may cause decreased alertness.

Rosemary

Although Rosemary has been used medicinally for many years, researchers are now proving that it isn't just folklore but that rosemary does contain many properties that make it a powerful all round treatment for many conditions. These complaints are varied ranging from Alzheimer's disease and other dementias all the way through to cancer and heart disease.

Several studies have shown that rosemary contains over 20 antioxidants. One of these, Rosmarinic acid whilst having antiviral, antibacterial and anti-inflammatory properties also protects the brain from the build up of amyloid plaques (and dissolves any build up already present) – one of the main causes of Alzheimer's. Rosmarinic acid also prevents the release of toxins from the amyloid itself which can cause further memory loss.

Rosemary extract also helps prevent the breakdown of acetylcholine one of the main neurotransmitters (or brain chemicals) involved in memory production and recall **(28)**.

As an aside, of all the rosemary compounds that slow the breakdown of acetylcholine several are easily absorbed through the skin, entering the blood stream and passing into the brain. Therefore, using a shampoo containing rosemary (which are readily available from health food stores or via the Internet) should in theory help preserve the amount of acetylcholine in the brain. The ancient Romans and Greeks used to wear laurels of rosemary in their hair to sharpen their brains – so maybe they knew something we have long since forgotten!

Whilst rosmarinic acid's properties are well documented with regard to supporting term memory, another recent study also showed that rosmarinic acid exerts a calming effect on the mind. This is an added bonus for anybody suffering the affects of Alzheimer's or dementia and researchers believe that the extract is especially effective for those suffering from mild to moderate Alzheimer's disease **(29)**.

Recommendation

A daily supplement of 800mg of Rosemary leaf may be beneficial in relieving the symptoms of Alzheimer's disease.

And Finally...
Some Of The Lesser Known Herbs
That Are Also Very Good...

Galantamine – The New All Rounder

Most of our modern medicines are based on traditional herbal remedies. Once something is found that is beneficial science isolates the actives ingredients or chemicals and then sets about mass-producing it.

This is excellent up to a point – the draw back is that by only picking out the part that you feel is therapeutic you may actually remove some of the other chemicals that are naturally present that reduce the negative aspects of the "drug". This means that you end up with a very potent medicine that is effective but one that comes at a cost due to its inherent side effects.

Galantamine is one such remedy.

Originally a compound isolated from several different plants (including the daffodil and common snow drop) and used as a remedy in its own right – mainly for physiotherapy treatments including muscular aches and pains, but also for wide ranging neurological (nerve), gastroenterological(stomach and gut) and cardiological (heart) purposes.

Galantamine, a cholinesterase inhibitor, has now been manufactured into a medication for Alzheimer's and vascular dementia. This is good in that it makes the treatment available from a medical doctor (the trade names for these drugs are Reminyl and Reminyl XL) but, unfortunately, it also means that the number of side effects has increased. These include feeling sick, vomiting, feeling dizzy, headaches, loss of appetite and, more importantly, an increased death rate was noted during the trials of galantamine for those patients that received it **(30)**.

However there is still good news.

Firstly, galantamine is still available as a herbal remedy on the internet and the herbal treatment has fewer side-effects than its pharmaceutical counterpart although it can still affect liver and kidney function – therefore caution needs to be taken if you wish to try this supplement and you suffer with any problem that affects these organs.

Secondly, the dosages that are required to produce significant changes in cognition and behaviour are quite small. Research has shown that the optimum dose for both tolerance and effectiveness is 16mg a day.

Thirdly, studies have shown the effectiveness of galantamine with patient's suffering mild to moderate Alzheimer's disease score more highly in memory and thinking tests when they take the supplement **(31, 32)**.

In addition to the greater cognition, doses of 16mg of galantamine also seemed to help sufferers not only look after themselves better but also have fewer emotional symptoms such as agitation, restlessness and aggression.

And as if that wasn't enough of the good stuff, galantamine has another distinct advantage over other drugs and even other herbal remedies. Galantamine is a cholinesterase inhibitor and as such it increases the amount of acetylcholine in the brain which as you know improves memory, thinking and rationalising.

But it also does two others thing…

Not only does it increase the amount of acetylcholine in the brain but also it binds to specific receptors on the nerves further stimulating their action. These receptors (in particularly nicotinic receptors) are known to enhance cerebral blood flow and cognitive and psychomotor functions **(33)**. And, although the action by which galantamine works is unclear it also seems to play a role in preventing nerve cell death **(34)**.

Recommendation

Galantamine has been associated with side effects that that range in severity. Consult your healthcare practitioner about whether galantamine is advisable for you.

A galantamine supplement of 16 mg a day can be beneficial. Suggested dose is 8mg in the morning and 8mg at night.

All in all, galantamine has many roles in the treatment of Alzheimer's disease, not all of which are fully understood – yet all are vital.

Myricetin

Myricetin is a flavonoid that is commonly found in foods such as berries, vegetables, teas, wine and herbs. Like the other flavonoids it has aroused considerable interest recently because of its potential beneficial effects on health – flavonoids have been reported to have antiviral, anti-allergic, anti-platelet, anti-inflammatory, anti-tumour and antioxidant activities. Research has shown that myricetin has many of these properties and although the exact mechanism is unclear, scientists in Japan have found that myricetin also has the ability to inhibit the accumulation of beta-amyloid protein (35).

In addition to preventing the build-up of amyloid deposits in the brain it also dissolved the amyloid deposits that had previously formed. It was also noted in the study that Myricetin may have the ability to detoxify the brain by removing heavy metals (this was particularly noted with iron) from the brain and therefore lower the risk of Alzheimer's disease that is associated with these deposits (36).

Myricetin can be purchased over the Internet and although higher dosages have been suggested for lowering cholesterol, I would recommend a daily dose of 100mg in the treatment of Alzheimer's.

<u>Vinpocetine</u>

Vinpocetine, an extract derived from the periwinkle plant *Vinca minor,* is also showing a number of nerve protecting properties that may help in the treatment of vascular dementia, Alzheimer's and other neurological disorders where oxidative stress may be involved. It is an antioxidant and vasodilator and has been shown to not only increase blood flow to the brain but also increase ATP production (or the production of energy) as well as increase glucose transport in the brain helping to increase cerebral activity.

Research has shown that it helps prevent oxidative stress in cells treated with amyloid, attenuate cognitive deficits, reduces ischaemia-induced hippocampal cell loss (i.e. it prevents cell death in the area of the brain that controls memory formation and storage) and increases blood flow to the brain and the way it uses glucose **(37)**.

It has been shown that a dose of up to 10 mg of Vinpocetine three times a day is safe in adults.

Although the compound proved not to cause birth defects it is not recommended for pregnant women because of the possibility of increased sensitivity in pregnancy. Therefore its use in women who are fertile should be interrupted in case of pregnancy.

Recommendation

10mg of Vinpocetine three times a day may be beneficial for those suffering from vascular dementia or Alzheimer's disease.

Ferulic Acid

Ferulic Acid is a phytochemical (i.e. a chemical that is found naturally in plants) and is found in a variety of foods especially cereals such as brown rice, wheat and oats. It is also found in coffee, apples, artichokes, peanuts, oranges and pineapple. The important thing about ferulic acid is that it is a powerful anti-inflammatory and antioxidant that has the ability to pass into the nerves of the brain neutralising free radicals (which could cause damage to cell membranes and DNA) and prevent amyloid build up.

Recent studies testing a derivative of Ferulic Acid (ferulic acid ethyl ester) have shown quite remarkable results in animal experiments and there is no reason to believe that these results should not be replicable in humans.

Researchers have shown that when gerbils have been given compounds of Ferulic acid in their water for only four weeks and then been injected with amyloid proteins they were protected from decreases in learning and memory function and other performance skills. Those that hadn't received the Ferulic acid all showed impairment in memory, performance and behaviour during testing **(38, 39)**. From these results the researchers concluded that long-term use of Ferulic acid induces resistance to amyloid toxicity in the brain which suggests that it may be a useful preventive against Alzheimer's and other oxidative stress-related neurodegenerative or nerve degenerating conditions.

Ferulic Acid is widely available as a supplement over the internet in dosages of up to 250mg and there are no known contra-indications.

Recommendation

A dose of 250 mg of ferulic acid may be beneficial in the treatment of Alzheimer's disease and other neurodegenerative disorders.

Ashwagandha

Ashwagandha holds a place in Ayurvedic (or Indian) medicine similar to the way ginseng does in Chinese medicine. Although its name is derived because its roots smell like a horse – "Ashwa" means "horse" and "Gandha" means "odour" - don't let this put you off!

It is a very potent herb that can play many roles in Alzheimer's and other dementias as it is a powerful rejuvenative herb and adaptogen (meaning it can help increase endurance whilst also helping to increase energy and strengthen the immune system). In addition to all of this, it also has anti-inflammatory, anti-stress properties and is a potent antioxidant with mind-boosting capabilities.

Ashwagandha contains flavonoids and many other active ingredients and it is the combination of these that are believed to account for Ashwagandha's many medicinal roles. Researchers from the University of Leipzig, Germany and also researchers in India have discovered that Ashwagandha increases acetylcholine receptor activity in the brain and it is this that partly explains its cognition and memory enhancing effects **(40)**.

Other researchers have also discovered that Ashwagandha stimulates the growth of human nerve cells and may play an important role in repairing damaged brain pathways in the ageing brain, whilst also preventing the loss of other brain nerves and synapses (or nerve connections).

This is vitally important as Ashwagandha can not only prevent brain damage but also repair damage that has already occurred **(41)**! This led the lead researcher to state that Withanolide-A (one of the active ingredients in Ashwagandha) is "an important candidate for the therapeutic treatment of neurodegenerative diseases, as it is able to reconstruct neuronal networks".

Ashwagandha is also a sedative and a mood enhancer and may also play a role in improving sleep and behaviour in those suffering from Alzheimer's or other forms of dementia.

The herb is readily available over the Internet in both a powdered form and as a tea, tincture or a capsule. Care must be taken however as its raw seeds can be toxic and because of this it should be prepared and used only as prescribed by an experienced practitioner.

Recommendation

I would recommend that you use this herb only as prescribed by your herbalist, health food stockist or general practitioner.

Huperzine

Huperzine A is a herbal extract from the Chinese moss Huperzia Serrata. Although it has a long history of use in Traditional Chinese Medicine for reducing pain, fever and inflammation, it is also commonly used as a diuretic, antispasmodic, and hemostyptic (a compound that reduces blood flow) as well as a herb known for its memory enhancing properties.

It is only recently that western science has turned its attention to this "wonder drug" as a therapeutic treatment for Alzheimer's and other memory loss disorders such as senile dementia and age-related cognitive decline as they have discovered that it can protect brain cells against amyloid plaques, glutamate, free radicals, reduced blood flow to the brain and nerve cell death **(42)**. What is more important is that it does all this without any major side-effects (although excessive dosages may cause headaches, nausea, vomiting and diarrhoea).

Huperzine A works by inhibiting the activity of the chemical that depletes the body of acetylcholine whilst actively creating more acetylcholine. This allows the neurotransmitter to work for longer and more efficiently and therefore increases cognition and brain function.

As already mentioned acetylcholine is an extremely important neurotransmitter as it enhances communication between nerve cells and is responsible for memory, concentration and focus and if it is broken down or destroyed too quickly it causes incomplete nerve firings and failure to send the correct messages between nerve cells.

The big advantage that Huperzine A has over the pharmaceutical drugs that aim to do the same thing is that it has fewer side-effects and its action is more powerful and longer lasting **(43)**!

Recommendation

One to two 50mcg capsules of Huperzine A daily will improve memory and may slow the progression of Alzheimer's disease and other dementias.

Because it has similar actions to other medications prescribed for Alzheimer's disease (for example tacrine, physostigmine and donepezil) you should consult your general practitioner before taking Huperzine A.

Any one suffering from high blood pressure should not take Huperzine A.

Bacopa Monniera or Brahmi

Bacopa monniera (or as it is more commonly known Brahmi) is a traditional Indian herbal remedy that has been used for centuries in Ayurvedic medicine as a "mind enhancer", it has been used to treat and help those affected by stroke, nervous breakdown, mental exhaustion, hyperactivity, anxiety, Parkinsons, Alzheimer's, epilepsy and aged related dementia.

The powerful benefits of Bacopa are showing no end and it is beneficial for all ages...

Initially, Bacopa was most commonly used in Asia amongst students to improve mental alertness, enhance learning and academic performance as it improves mental acuity and clarity (i.e. it allows you to become focussed on one topic without your mind wandering) whilst also improving your ability to remember things for longer and with less stress!

Since the 60's various studies have been conducted to test its safety and toxicity and the results have been unanimous. Without exception the research has proved "that this standardised extract improves protein activity and protein synthesis, especially in the brain cells" and studies carried out in normal healthy children, elderly subjects with age associated memory impairment and children with attention deficit hyperactivity disorder have declared Bacopa to be a safe, well tolerated and effective treatment – all without side-effects.

Recent studies have also focused on Bacopa's effectiveness in treating depression with promising results. It has been used successfully to treat the symptoms associated with depression (it calms the mind and promotes relaxation whilst decreasing anxiety and restlessness) without any of the side-effects that are often associated with drugs such as Prozac, Paxil, and Zoloft. The interesting thing about Bacopa is that whilst calming and sedating it doesn't cause drowsiness or dull the mind further like prescribed sedatives can.

Also, Bacopa is a powerful natural free radical scavenger (100mg of Bacopa has 5 time the potency of the recommended daily allowance of vitamin E) whilst also increasing the activity of other antioxidant compounds. It is this activity of Bacopa that is believed to be behind some of its memory enhancing properties as studies have shown it targeting and protecting the memory centres of the brain such as the hippocampus (where memories are formed) and the frontal cortex (which expresses them) even more effectively than conventionally prescribed drugs.

Recommendation

400-500mg of Bacopa extract daily should prove beneficial for all cognitive disorders.
Bacopa has no known contraindications or side effects.

Wormwood – It's very good!

Researchers have reported that wormwood extract has the ability to stimulate specific brain chemicals and may have a beneficial effect on serious age-related brain disorders like Alzheimer's disease.

Wormwood is renowned for its distinct bitter taste which is why the ancient Romans gave it the name *absinthium* meaning bitter and one of its early uses was as flavouring – particularly (and not surprisingly!) in absinthe. The old Anglo-Saxon word *wermode* means "mind preserver" – which seems fitting given its brain-boosting properties.

Wormwood is a rich source of essential oils all of which are responsible for its memory-boosting benefits and back in 2000, researchers from the U.K. conducted a study to evaluate whether there was any basis to these claims and mixed wormwood extract with human brain cells...

What they found was that the extracts were able to bind to the outside membrane of the cells responsible for memory and learning (44) and stimulate them to work at a higher level and thus improve memory.

Another study tested over 20 medicinal plants (including wormwood and ginseng) for their ability to stimulate the brain and in particular nerve growth factors (the chemicals needed for nerves to repair themselves and grow). When the plants were studied they found that wormwood extract was able to stimulate the production of nerve growth factors thereby encouraging normal brain cell function.

Based on these findings, the researchers claim that wormwood extract may be useful in fighting serious age-related brain disorders such as Parkinson's and Alzheimer's disease (45)

Further research from Denmark reported that wormwood extract has the ability to stimulate a specific brain neurotransmitter.

In patients with Alzheimer's disease, a chemical called GABA becomes deficient and this has been found to contribute to the memory loss which is characteristic of the disease. However, extracts of wormwood have the ability to boost the production of GABA in the brain and have an overall positive effect on memory (**46**).

I would recommend a starting dose of 500mg of wormwood (in capsule form) 3 times a day. Should you prefer you can make a wormwood tea (however this is an acquired taste!) by steeping 2.5 -5 grams of wormwood in hot water and drinking 3 cups a day. I would not recommend the use of wormwood essential oil unless under the supervision of a trained healthcare practitioner or herbalist.

Wormwood can cause mild stomach upset but this is extremely rare when it is taken at the recommended dose. There are no known contraindications although I would not recommend it is taken during pregnancy or by people with severe liver or kidney disease.

And finally, a supplement that everybody should be taking regardless of whether they feel they need it or not...

Phosphatidylserine (PS)

Phosphatidylserine or PS for short has been called "the single best means for conserving memory and other higher brain functions" by one of the world's experts in nutrition Dr. Parris Kidd in his book "Phosphatidylserine (PS): Number One Brain Booster".

Dr. Thomas Crook author of "The Memory Cure" has also stated that "PS is by far the best of all the drugs and nutritional supplements we have ever tested for retarding Age Associated Memory Impairment (AAMI)"

So with those two heavy-weights behind this miracle nutrient I believe we should waste no more time and dive right in to its amazing properties…

Phosphatidylserine is a nutrient that is 100% natural, is completely safe and there are no reported side-effects or adverse reactions. It is most heavily concentrated in the membranes of brain cells where it plays an important role in controlling the transmission of information from one cell to another, cell repair and renewal as well as the manufacture and release of neurotransmitters (brain chemicals) which are necessary for the nerves to work correctly and vital for memory storage.

PS is not classed as an essential fatty acid as the body can make it. Unfortunately, making it is complicated and because it is found in relatively limited supply in food (some natural sources of PS are green leafy vegetables, fish, rice, soy products, eggs, organ meats and brain!) it is not readily obtained from the diet – hence the need for supplementation is important, particularly as we age.

Taken as a supplement PS is quickly absorbed into the blood where it can enter the brain and start producing the neurotransmitters adrenalin, noradrenalin, serotonin and dopamine. However it doesn't just affect these four neurotransmitters, because it also enhances the performance of cell membranes it improves the action of all neurotransmitters.

Whilst in the body PS also acts to increase the transportation of nutrients into the cells of the brain and helps eliminate waste products. This is important because as we age our cells become overloaded with cholesterol, hydrogenated and "trans" fats which alters their ability to absorb vital nutrients and produce the required energy to function efficiently.

PS can help improve virtually every function of the brain and body various studies have shown that it has a significant impact on:

Improving memory,
Improving concentration and recall,
Improving mood and personality,
Improving the ability to perform activities of daily living,
Helping the body adapt to stress – both physical and mental, Improving attention deficit (ADD) and hyperactivity,
Improving recovery after exercise.

In some research studies PS has been known to restore up to 14 years' worth of memory function in subjects with abnormally accelerated memory decline and most studies of PS are encouraging regardless of the level of memory impairment. In more than 35 trials on human subjects (over a period of 30 years or more) all show that PS is important for brain function. Sixteen or so trials have indicated that learning, memory, vocabulary and concentration all show signs of improvement whilst others have shown that it improves mood, sociability and alertness.

To validate some of these claims I would like to share with you the results of a couple research studies into the effects of PS on Alzheimer's disease...

A study performed in 1987 in Italy with patients diagnosed with early Alzheimer's showed that supplementation with 300mg a day of PS for 60 days produced a statistically significant benefit on delayed memory recollection (**47**).

In 1988 another group of Italian researchers supplemented a group of patients with 200mg a day of PS for 3 months. These subjects were then assessed over a two year period and compared with a similar group of patients that had not received PS supplementation. It was found that the differences after 3 and 6 months were significant both with personal memory, overall memory and performance of everyday activities – with those given the placebo deteriorating considerably whilst those given the PS having improved (**48**).

Whilst the body can make some PS itself we generally need to rely on supplementation to keep ourselves at an adequate level (especially if vegetarian as the majority of the PS that we consume comes from organ meats), and there are different sources of PS that are available in supplement form and each one is slightly different in potency and effectiveness.

PS can be derived from vegetable extracts (e.g. white cabbage), bovine sources and soy based products. The vegetable based PS seems to be the least effective and with doubts about bovine products (with the resultant BSE or "Mad Cow Disease" scares) most PS is produced from soy. Various studies have tested the effectiveness of soy based PS and all of them have found that it is as good if not slightly better in reversing age related memory loss than the other forms.

Whichever source of PS you decide upon you can rest assured knowing that there have never been any recorded side-effects and it will not react with any medication.

Phosphatidylserine has been shown to be effective in both slowing and reversing age related memory loss and early stage Alzheimer's, and for these reasons I feel that it should be a staple in everyone's fight against dementia. I would recommend a daily dose of 300 mg for at least three months (taking a dose of 100mg three times a day) in order to build up your reserves and saturate you body. After this you could drop to a maintenance dose of no less than 100mg of PS a day depending on your age and severity of mental decline. There is no evidence that a permanent dose of 300mg has any adverse effect but if you are solely using it for a preventative measure and / or are still in your early to mid 40's then 100mg should be sufficient.

A couple of words of caution however before you rush out to buy it (and you know you should!)...

Firstly, it is also possible to buy phosphorylated serine – **this is not the same thing**, it doesn't have the same health benefits and it can cause uncomfortable adverse reactions.

Secondly, most nutritional supplements of PS only contain about 20% phosphatidylserine – the rest is usually other phospholipids or essential fatty acids. For this reason you will need to check the labels to see how much PS you are actually getting and increase the dosage accordingly – even if this means taking up to 5 times the suggested dose to get you up to 100-300mg a day!

Some researchers suggest that just taking PS alone can have a dramatic effect of reversing dementia and cognitive decline and I would agree – but just think how effective it could be if you incorporated it into a new health regime! I have talked already about changes you

can make to diet and lifestyle, supplements you can take that have a known effect but just think what you could to if you combined 2, 3 or more of the techniques you have learnt already.

Recommendation

I would recommend PS as a staple nutrient both for treating Alzheimer's and dementia but also for use in preventing it.
I would recommend a daily dose of 300 mg for at least three months (taking 100mg three times a day) in order to build up your reserves. After this you could drop to a maintenance dose of 100mg

---

Section
Five

The Effects of Drinking Water on Alzheimer's - and the effect of not!

All complementary and alternative therapies place tremendous store on drinking water and the role that it plays in maintaining optimum health and illness prevention.

Now it looks as if they are being proved right!

In fact one of the main therapies that I both practice and teach, Total Body Modification, (you can contact www.tbmseminars.com for more information and to find a practitioner near you) advocates drinking one litre of water for every 24 kilos (or fraction of) that you weigh. This is because all of the systems of the body require an adequate supply of water to function at their most efficient – especially if you are toxic or suffering from the effects of heavy metal poisoning. The easiest way to remember this and for it to strike home is realise that the "the *solution* to *pollution* is *dilution*"

But now it is coming to light that the type of water that you drink is also important in controlling and reducing your risk of Alzheimer's. A recent study found that drinking mineral water rich in silicon is a natural way to reduce the amount of aluminium in people suffering with Alzheimer's (and before there is uproar that there is no scientific proof that aluminium causes Alzheimer's there is scientific proof that all sufferers of Alzheimer's disease have consistently higher levels of aluminium in their blood).

This study showed that in eight out of ten patients that drank 1 and a ½ litres of mineral water a day for five days showed a reduction in their levels of aluminium.

This is important to note for two reasons;

1, Silicon is a natural protector against aluminium toxicity and may account for some of the decline, but also
2, Municipal (or tap) water often has fluoride added to it and this is a binding agent for aluminium and therefore helps it to get absorbed into the body – thereby increasing its concentration.

The aluminium concentration of water is also increased when certain cookware is used so this should also be taken into account (– but I will be cover this in the section on aluminium and Alzheimer's).

One final nudge to make you reach for the water rather than your favourite beverage is that sugary drinks have been linked to an increase in Alzheimer's.

A study reported from the American Society for Biochemistry and Molecular Biology suggests that drinks with a high sugar content have been linked to the increase in risk of Alzheimer's. This study found that mice that were fed a 10% sugar solution showed a decline in learning and memory retention, and their brains contained over twice as many amyloid plaque deposits – a hallmark of Alzheimer's – as those not given the sugary drink.

How much is a 10% sugar solution in human terms you may be asking, and that is a good question.

Roughly, it is the equivalent to 5 cans of carbonated drink consumed on a daily basis (an amount you may think is hard to achieve) but there are other ways to reach this total without trying too hard as we consume about 20% of our calories through drinks including alcohol, sports drinks and fruit juices.

The other thing to consider is that because mice have a high metabolic rate they can therefore "burn" off this sugar overload more easily than we do so the number of drinks needed to reach this overload may actually be less in humans!

Recommendation

Drink at least two litres of mineral water a day.

Fit a water filter to remove heavy metals and fluoride.

Heavy Metal Is Bad For You
(and I don't just mean the music!)

For many years it has been known that heavy metal poisoning is not only detrimental to physical health but mental health as well – but now more and more research is driving this point home.

When considering mental health and cognition it was always considered that aluminium played the greatest role in causing the symptoms related to Alzheimer's and other dementias. However this is no longer the case and for this reason, this section is going to look at not only aluminium but also zinc, copper and mercury.

So let's begin...

Aluminium and Alzheimer's

There can be very little doubt left that aluminium certainly aggravates but may also cause the symptoms of Alzheimer's (as well as cell death) – particularly when combined with the protein that causes plaque formation in the brain. The Canadian Journal of Public Health has shown that Alzheimer's sufferers have much higher levels of aluminium in their brains than "normal" patients **(1)**.

The question is where does it come from and what can you do about it?

There are two main sources of aluminium that you are likely to come into contact with – both on a daily basis and I bet you haven't given either much thought!

The first is your drinking water.

Now, I know we have touched on this earlier but a study from the University of California has found a direct link between the levels of aluminium in the water and Alzheimer's. The group focused on an area of Italy noted

147

for its higher than average occurrence of the disease and discovered that their water supply had unusually high concentrations of aluminium – in some cases up to six times the amount recommended as being safe!

Unfortunately nearly all sources of public drinking water contain traces of aluminium and this is aggravated by the presence of fluoride alongside it (put there for its own dubious health benefits). It may be just coincidence that the world's most fluoridated country, Ireland, has a massive 30,000 cases of Alzheimer's out of a total population of three million.

Other areas where there is a high level of aluminium (regardless of the addition of fluoride) are Scotland and North of England (particularly Northumberland, Tyne and Wear and Durham) and Cornwall according to a study by Southampton University of 80 districts of England and Wales funded by the Medical Research Council (1989).

In these areas the incidence of Alzheimer's was 1½ times higher than elsewhere and the concentration of aluminium in these areas water supplies was up to 5 times the European Communities level that is deemed safe. Because the aluminium found in tap water is chemically different from the aluminium that the body absorbs from food this has led certain water companies to remove the aluminium from their water treatment processes.

The other source to consider is from your cooking utensils.

Not only does the presence of fluoride increase the rate of aluminium that is released from the cookware but it also increases the amount of it that can get absorbed by the body – fluoride can increase the rate of absorption of aluminium into your system by up to 800 percent! This combination of aluminium fluoride has also been shown to cross the blood-brain barrier.

This was something that was previously thought not to occur but recent tests conducted at Duke University in North Carolina have confirmed that it does. The results from the research carried out there suggest that this combination of aluminium and fluoride in water **can** result in pre-senile dementia and also kidney damage **(2)**.

At home this source is easy to avoid – just don't use aluminium cookware (use stainless steel or cast iron) and don't cook with aluminium foil if at all possible. Also, non stick pans (such as Teflon and Tefal) are made from a fluoride containing polymer which releases fluoride when heated **(3)**. It may be harder to avoid when eating out as most professional cookware (as I have been led to believe) is aluminium based – something to do with quick and uniform heat distribution – but at least you can reduce the risk at home.

You can reduce the risk further if you use bottled mineral water or install a water filter that will remove the fluoride from your tap water. Now, I realise that this is an effort, the filters may be hard to find and you may have to install it etc. but it is worth the effort as aluminium doesn't get released from cookware without fluoride present.

Other sources of aluminium that you may wish to limit your exposure to are cosmetics, antiperspirants and antacids. If you read the "ingredients" you will always find one or two aluminium compounds listed. If you want to remove this possible source from your environment (and still keep your friends!) I would recommend switching to a deodorant (where there is less aluminium if any) or changing to an antiperspirant crystal / stone that you can purchase over the internet.

Recommendation

Avoid aluminium cookware, packaging and canned foods as much as possible.

Change your antiperspirant to a deodorant.

To help detox the body of aluminium I would suggest contacting your healthcare professional or using one of the many detox systems that are available.

I personally prefer the detox process recommended by Total Body Modification (www.tbmseminars.com) but I would also suggest supplementation with malic acid and magnesium. A1000mg of malic acid will help to eliminate the aluminium from the body and 250-500mg of magnesium will help to block its re-absorption. Magnesium can cause a loosening of the stool and an increase in bowel movement so use this up to a level that you can tolerate and again consult you healthcare provider before starting or changing supplements.

> ### Recommendation
>
> Think about having a heavy metal detox.
>
> A malic acid supplement of 1000mg a day can be beneficial.

<u>Magnesium</u>

Whilst we are discussing Magnesium, a study conducted by the Massachusetts Institute of Technology has shown that magnesium also helps to regulate the brain receptors that play a crucial role in learning and memory. Their research shows that a deficiency of magnesium contributes to an impaired ability to learn and memorize, while an abundance of magnesium may actually boost cognitive function by enhancing the neuroplasticity (or the way nerves change and adapt) of nerve synapses – the connections between brain cells – preventing cognitive decline and memory degeneration.

> ### Recommendation
>
> A magnesium supplement of 250-500mg a day can be beneficial. (Supplement to bowel tolerance).

Although I have covered aluminium in detail there are other metals that have been linked to Alzheimer's and dementia....

Some of the latest research shows that there may be a "new kid on the block" that is equally as bad if not worse and it goes by the name of mercury!

Mercury Madness

Some of the most recent has looked into the effects of mercury and the findings are not good.

A team of medical researchers from the University of Kentucky have been looking at the problem of mercury in Alzheimer's patients for many years. In fact, their findings have led them to conclude that *"there is increasing evidence that mercury, rather than aluminium is the highest trace element found in the brains of Alzheimer's disease victims."*

Their research has consistently shown that there are higher levels of mercury in the brains of Alzheimer's sufferers according to autopsy findings than any other trace metal. This has led them to state that "the present study suggests that the elevation of mercury in Alzheimer's disease is the most important of the imbalances we have observed." **(4)**

They are not alone in this view.

Their work has been supported by other researchers. A team reporting their findings in the Federation of American Societies for Experimental Biology in the early 1990's confirmed that mice fed with a diet rich in mercury showed diminished tubulin levels

152

similar to those of Alzheimer's patients. Tubulin is important because it is a protein necessary for forming nerve fibres and without it the brain creates tangled nerve connections that distort and reduce the messages that the brain sends.

This study was also important in showing that mice fed with a diet high in aluminium alone failed to create these nerve tangles as the levels of tubulin remained unaltered. This led the team to conclude that "certain complex forms of mercury must be considered as a potential source of the aetiology of Alzheimer's disease." **(5)**

There are however another couple of ideas on the role of heavy metals in relation to Alzheimer's disease.

The first suggests that it is not caused by an individual heavy metal but rather an accumulation of many that are causative agents. Studies have suggested that it is a build up of mercury in the tissues of the brain that predisposes the brain to an accumulation of aluminium

Other theories suggest that it may actually be a deficiency in certain trace minerals that leads to a build up of both mercury and aluminium. For example, the brains of Alzheimer's sufferers are often depleted in both zinc and selenium – both of which are known to offer a protective role against heavy metal toxicity in all body tissues.

Another idea is that it is neither mercury nor aluminium that are the cause of the changes that are found in the brain of sufferers – but that they accumulate because of changes that are already taking place **(6)**. This means that if is down to disease and alterations already taking place in the brain and other tissues that allows these toxins to accumulate and be deposited at these sites **(4)** and not the toxins causing the disease.

From a personal viewpoint because both aluminium and mercury are known to be neurotoxins (i.e. they kill nerve cells) I would urge caution and limit exposure to these metals as much as possible.

So the question now is how do you avoid mercury?

Although it is impossible to say how mercury gets into the brain it is possible to limit your exposure to it. The main accredited source is from amalgam fillings. Studies have shown that mercury and other heavy metals can be released as a vapour from these fillings when chewing food, grinding your teeth or even just through cleaning them vigorously! These studies indicate that approximately two thirds of all the mercury found in the body is from dental amalgam and that it can remain there for up to forty years.

It is possible to have the fillings removed by specialist dentists but the mercury can also leach away from the fillings and into the teeth and gums – making it hard to fully remove all of its presence.

There is however a couple of simple techniques you can use that will limit this leakage (and you can do these yourself at home). Either rub along the jaw line and the area of the teeth of the outside of the cheek with a tape head demagnetiser (available over the internet – originally used to stop the old ferrous oxide tapes sticking to the reels in tape players and tangling up). If you do this for about thirty seconds each side of the face this will be enough to prevent a problem.

Or you can use a magnet and with the north side of the magnet on the outside of the cheek shine a torch though the open mouth and onto the filled teeth that are in front of the magnet. Do this for about ten seconds per filling and you will notice an improvement. Both of these techniques are from Total Body Modification and work well until your next dental visit after which you just repeat the process.

The other major source of mercury is from fish and sea food products and the larger the fish the greater the problem. In the United States the F.D.A. (Food and Drug Administration) has warned of the risks of eating tuna, salmon, mackerel and swordfish whilst pregnant because of the possible risks to the developing foetus. It makes you wonder if it is such a risk during pregnancy why isn't it a risk at any other time?

Recommendation
Consider if it is practical to remove any amalgam fillings.
Consider treating your fillings yourself using the techniques described above.
Limit your intake of tuna, salmon and mackerel.
Consider a heavy metal detox.

Because I briefly touched on the role of selenium and zinc and the effects that a deficiency may have on the body it is worth covering them in a little more detail here.

<u>Selenium</u>

Selenium is an essential trace mineral which functions primarily as a powerful anti-oxidant preventing free radical damage to cells. Low levels of selenium are associated with a higher risk of cancer, cardiovascular disease, immune deficiencies and premature ageing.

However, a study published in the American Journal of Epidemiology **(7)** has shown how dietary intake is also related to cognition and memory retention. The study lasting over two years found that long term those subjects that had lower levels of selenium performed poorer on cognitive testing. When correlated against those with the highest levels of selenium the difference in performance was equivalent to a staggering ten years difference in cognitive scores.

The lead author in the study stated that "selenium exposure, unlike other factors studied for Alzheimer's disease, is a factor that is easily modifiable by changing dietary habits or through supplements" but added that "long-term exposure to selenium may be needed to impact brain function later in life" – so best start now!

Like all supplements toxicity can occur at too high a daily dosage, but a range of 200-400 mcg daily is considered quite safe. I usually recommend a standard dose of 200mcg a day.

Recommendation

A selenium supplement of 200-400mcg a day can be beneficial in the prevention of Alzheimer's disease and dementia.

Why You Need To Think About Zinc

Zinc is a very strange supplement when used in the treatment of Alzheimer's disease. Too little and it will have no effect and too much and it may actually aggravate the condition – therefore balance is the key.

Although zinc is an essential trace element in human biology it is neurotoxic (poisonous to nerves) at high concentrations. Several studies have shown that high levels aggravate plaque formation actually causing more aggregations (or clumping of these plaques and nerve fibres) that are typically found in Alzheimer's patients.

Other studies however, have shown that the level of zinc found in the brains of those suffering from the condition are reduced particularly in the area of the hippocampus – the part related to memory and learning. Supplementation of 10 patient's suffering with Alzheimer's with zinc aspartate / sulphate showed significant improvements in their condition **(8, 9)**.

Other theories believe that it may be an imbalance of trace metals that allows a toxic overload of heavy metals to build up creating these changes in the brain. An important study **(10)** shows how they believe it is low general levels of zinc and selenium that cause a toxic build-up of heavy metals in the brain (particularly mercury) as they are its chief mineral antagonists (i.e. they block its absorption) and are known to have a protective role against heavy metal toxicity.

However, a yet unpublished study from 1991 showed that dosages of 90mg a day caused a decline in cognition after only 5 days.

Because of this uncertainty I would urge caution with the use of zinc supplements and limit the daily supplementation to 50mg of zinc a day and I would also consider undergoing a detox program to remove excess heavy metals from the system.

It is also important to note that the supplementation of zinc also needs to be combined with copper in a ratio of 10:1 (therefore 25mg zinc to 2.5mg copper) to enhance the correct metabolism.

> ### Recommendation
>
> A zinc supplement of no more than 50mg a day can be beneficial.

As I have briefly touched on supplementation with copper to enhance the effects of any zinc supplements taken it is worth looking at copper alone as it also plays a role in Alzheimer's. Unfortunately its role is almost as controversial as that of zinc.

<u>Copper and Cognition</u>

Whilst copper is essential for brain development, too much copper in the bloodstream may block the body's ability to rid itself of proteins that form the plaques found clogging the brains of Alzheimer's patients **(11)** and too little may increase the risk of mental decline **(12)**.

But again both of these studies need to be viewed with caution.

It may be that (as we touched on earlier) there are already disease processes that are going on in the brain that makes the elimination of copper harder and therefore it builds up. There may be other dietary factors involved that led to the build up. The first study was based on findings from rabbits fed a diet high in cholesterol (not their natural diet) and water that was laced with copper and therefore it makes extrapolating the results to a human population harder. Also, although there are traces of copper found in tap water (another reason to drink mineral water!) the number of plaques formed by the rabbits was much rarer in those drinking the copper laced liquid alone.

The other study which was based on humans (to spare the mice, rabbits and gerbils for a change!) showed that there was a direct correlation between higher levels of blood copper and greater cognition. Patients with higher blood copper levels make fewer mistakes in memory tests leading the researchers to remark that an increased uptake of dietary copper may be therapeutically relevant in the treatment of Alzheimer's disease.

Because of the uncertainty in the role copper plays in dementia I would recommend limiting the daily dosage to no more than 3mg a day.

Recommendation
A copper supplement of no more than 3mg a day can be beneficial.

Before I finish the section on heavy metals I would like to cover one more metal that has implications in the progression of Alzheimer's disease and that is the controversial role of iron.

Alzheimer's and an "Iron Will"?

Before I start I must state my views on iron supplements so that everything is "above board"...

I only recommend iron supplementation in the most extreme cases of anaemia for two reasons. Firstly the body tends not to lose a great amount of iron and it has no known mechanism for getting rid of any excess. In cases of iron deficiency / anaemia there is usually always a cause that should be initially treated before any supplementation is started. These causes are usually stomach ulcers, severe haemorrhoids or other undetected bleeding and these should be found and corrected first. Excess iron has a very strong oxidative role in the body i.e. it promotes ageing and free radical damage and therefore, I believe, should be treated with caution.

Using new MRI techniques researchers have discovered that Alzheimer's sufferers have an iron build up or deposits in the brain **(13)**. Although high iron levels and free radical damage have been linked with a variety of neurological disorders such as Parkinson's and Huntington's disease (as well as heart disease and certain cancers) the lead researcher in this study believes that there is also an extremely strong association with Alzheimer's.

However, other researchers believe that it may be a deficiency of iron that makes the body go into overdrive and produce too much destructive heme (an iron compound) to compensate. They believe that it is therefore vital to have enough iron in your system to start with **(14)**, and that supplementation with iron and other essential vitamins (particularly the B vitamins that we covered earlier) may play an important role in slowing the disease.

Although the safe upper limit of iron supplementation has been set at 45mg per day I would feel hesitant to take more than 10mg a day particular if you have any degenerative conditions such as those listed previously, if you are post menopausal, suffer from high blood pressure, high cholesterol or diabetes.

Recommendation

Sometimes supplementation with iron is necessary but there may be other treatments available.

I would advise caution and if possible set a limit at 10mg of iron supplementation a day.

Get More From Boron

Boron has been linked with improvements in bone, mineral and lipid metabolism, energy utilization and immune function – and it is vital that all of these are kept at an optimum in combating the ageing process.

However, there is another important system of the body that boron is now been recognised as of vital importance to – and that is the brain and nervous system.

Evidence from a review of five studies from the United States Department of Agriculture's Human Nutrition Centre where they reviewed the electrical activity of the brains of both animals and humans have conclusively shown that diminished levels boron result in decreased brain activity resulting in a poorer performance on tasks of motor speed and dexterity, attention and short-term memory.

It has been previously believed that a good, well-balanced diet would provide an adequate daily supply of boron, but the studies found that supplementation with 3.75 mg of the mineral improved brain function even more. Lower levels of boron were found in those subjects that performed significantly poorer in tasks that required manual dexterity, eye and hand coordination, attention, perception, short-term memory and long-term memory – leading the researcher to conclude that boron "is important for brain and psychological function in humans".

Although, there have been no studies that show any toxicity with boron, I would restrict a daily dosage to less than 5mg.

Recommendation

A supplement of no greater than 5mg of boron may be of benefit in improving memory and cognition.

The Low Down on Lithium

Some readers may already be aware that lithium is a very useful treatment for certain mental illnesses. However fewer readers may know that there are different types of lithium compounds available and that the prescribed type is just one of them.

The lithium salts that this section will deal with are used in very small doses and their effects have been linked with slowing the progression of Parkinson's disease, senile dementia and more importantly Alzheimer's disease.

Lithium has three important roles to play in protecting the brain. Firstly studies have shown that it can actually increase the size of the brain (this counteracts the natural shrinkage that occurs with age) by slowing cell and also by promoting cell growth **(15)**. Secondly it offers protection against toxins and thirdly helps form proteins that further protect the brain.

With Alzheimer's sufferers lithium's role becomes even more important. It has a role in preventing the build up of amyloid proteins that form the plaques which are the signature of Alzheimer's disease **(16)**. It also chelates heavy metals (particularly aluminium) so that they can be more easily removed from the body. In fact one researcher believes that lithium remains one of the most potent chelators that we have at our disposal for removing aluminium from the body **(17)**.

The lithium salts that I recommend are far more easily absorbed by the cells of the body than those prescribed pharmaceutically. These supplements are lithium orotate or lithium aspartate (usually orotate) and the dose that I suggest patients take is to start off on 5mg a day and then to build it up to no more than 20mg over several weeks.

At dosages of 20mg per day there are very rarely any side effects (as this is 10-20 times lower than the pharmaceutical dose) and a lot to gain.

Recommendation

A lithium orotate or aspartate supplement may be beneficial in protecting the brain and preventing further damage.

Build up slowly to a dosage of no more than 20mg a day.

Section
Six

Summary of Possible Actions To Take

There has been a lot of information presented to you in this book – so much so that it may appear a little daunting! For that reason I want to précis a lot of the material into bite size pieces that you can contemplate and act on with ease should you so wish.

In order to do this I am going to break down the various treatment approaches that you now have at hand into various sections for those of you that want to tackle a specific area at one time. Some readers may feel, for example, that changing lifestyle first may offer the best benefits, other may feel that reducing homocysteine or improving the levels of neurotransmitters may offer the best way forward for them – which ever you feel is best for you and your situation you will find the information summarised over the next few pages.

Remember that this will only be a summary of the things that you can implement to improve those various areas and I advise you to refer back to the main book for full information about any of the supplements or guidelines mentioned here.

For Those That Want To Treat Alzheimer's Disease and Dementia Though Changing Their Life Style.

1. **Stay Mentally Fit and Active.**

Consider taking up a hobby from the following categories:

- Music and Films – Watching nostalgic films and musicals, singing, playing "Name that Tune" etc.
- Craft and Hobby Activities – Playing cards, board games, word games or puzzles, knitting, woodwork etc.
- Cooking activities.
- Outdoor trips and visits
- Helping around the home.

2. **Stay Physically Fit and Active.**

- 15 minutes of exercise, three times a week ranging from the following activities – walking, hiking, bicycling, aerobics or callisthenics, swimming, water aerobics, weight training or stretching have all been shown to improve dementia and Alzheimer's disease.
- 20 minutes of housework has been shown to improve Alzheimer's and dementia.

3. Consider reducing the amount you smoke.

Unless you have the genes that predispose you to Alzheimer's disease (in which case smoking will have no effect on the chances of you developing the disease), the risk of developing Alzheimer's disease is increased by 2.3 times if you smoke.

4. Consider reducing the amount of alcohol you drink.

- Excessive alcohol consumption (three or more drinks daily) can lead to a decline in cognition and alcohol related dementia.
- Drink either **green, black, Rooibos or Oolong tea, fruit (especially grape) or vegetable juices.**

5. Reduce the volume of food and the amount of carbohydrates that you eat.

- Being over weight or having a large stomach increases your risk of all types of dementia.
- The greater your calorific intake is the greater your chances of dementia.
- Reducing or restricting your carbohydrate intake can halt or even reverse the symptoms of Alzheimer's disease especially if you have a gluten allergy.

6. Maintain an ideal blood sugar level.

If you are diabetic make sure that this is as accurately controlled as possible. Consider a daily supplement of **200mcg of Chromium Picolinate** (or **Chromium GTF**) to help regulate your blood sugar levels.

7. Consider a Mediterranean style diet.

- A Mediterranean diet is abundant in virgin olive oil, high quantities of fruit, vegetables, nuts and seeds, fish and wholegrain pulses and cereals.

8. Cut artificial sweeteners out of your diet.

9. Drink at least two litres of mineral water a day and / or fit a water filter to remove heavy metals and fluoride from your domestic water supply.

10. Reduce your exposure to Aluminium and Mercury.

- Avoid aluminium cookware, packaging and canned foods as much as possible.
- Change your antiperspirant to a deodorant.
- Consider working on your fillings to prevent mercury leakage.
- Think about having a heavy metal detox.

For Those That Want To Treat Alzheimer's Disease and Dementia
Though An Improvement In The Blood Supply To Their Brain.

1. **Control your Hypertension.**

   - Consider a daily supplement of **500mg of garlic** three times a day, **100mg of Co-enzyme Q10** and **1000mg to 1200 mg of hawthorn extract**.
   - Consider taking up gentle exercise two to three times a week.
   - Lose weight if necessary.

2. **Reduce your levels of Atherosclerosis**

   - Consider a daily supplement of **200mcg of Chromium Picolinate** (or **Chromium GTF**) to help prevent and reverse atherosclerosis and coronary artery disease
   - A daily supplement of **150 grams of whole oat products and 30 grams of barley bran** may help lower your risk of atherosclerosis and reduce you total cholesterol (and LDL cholesterol) in particular.

   - A daily dose of **12mg of Inositol** divided into 6 equal doses may be of benefit may be beneficial in reducing atherosclerosis.

3. Control your Diabetes.

- If you are diabetic make sure that this is as accurately controlled as possible.
- **Consider a supplement of Chromium Picolinate** or **Chromium GTF** (as mentioned above) to help regulate your blood sugar levels.
- A daily dose of up to **300mg vitamin B6** may help to prevent the development of insulin-dependent diabetes mellitus (consult your general practitioner before taking any niacin supplement if you suffer from ulcers, adult onset diabetes, liver disease or gout).

4. Control your Cholesterol.

Consider a daily supplement of **200i.u. to 400i.u. of vitamin E** and **250mg of Arjuna** to reduce your cholesterol.

5. Control your levels of Homocysteine.

Consider supplementing your diet with the following vitamins **B6, B12 and folic acid, eating plenty of cereals and green leafy vegetables** to lower your homocysteine level. A good starting point is **1 - 5mg of folic acid** (in severe cases of increased homocysteine), **50mg to 100mg of vitamin B6** (depending on severity) and **1mg of sub-lingual vitamin B12**. Also a daily supplement of **2g of Betaine HCl** may be beneficial in reducing homocysteine.

6. **Control your Irregular Heart Beat.**

It is possible to improve an irregular heart beat by:

- Controlling your cholesterol,
- Controlling your blood pressure,
- Maintaining your correct blood sugar levels (and diabetes if present),
- Do not drink more than two alcoholic drinks per day.
- Stop smoking.
- Control your weight and / or lose weight if necessary, and
- Get regular exercise – 20-30 minutes 2-3 times a week.

7. **Reduce the amount that you smoke.**

Unless you have the genes that predispose you to Alzheimer's disease (in which case smoking will have no effect on the chances of you developing the disease), the risk of developing Alzheimer's disease is increased by 2.3 times if you smoke.

8. **Control the amount of alcohol that you drink.**

Excessive alcohol consumption (three or more drinks daily) can lead to a decline in cognition and alcohol related dementia, however moderate drinking (one to three alcoholic drinks a day) may reduce the risk of vascular dementia (dementia caused by a series of small strokes) by 70%.

9. A daily dose of **2500-3000mg of vitamin C** and up to **800mg of vitamin E** may prove beneficial in improving blood flow, reducing atherosclerosis and reducing cholesterol.

10. Researchers have found that **50mg of Beta-Carotene** given on alternate days proved beneficial in decreasing cardiovascular disease.

11. A **Ginkgo Biloba supplement of up to 200mg a day** can be beneficial in thinning the blood and dilating blood vessels.

- Caution is advised if taking aspirin or other medications to thin the blood.

12. **10mg of Vinpocetine** three times a day may be beneficial for those suffering from vascular dementia or Alzheimer's disease.

For Those That Want To Treat Alzheimer's Disease and Dementia Though Reducing Their Homocysteine.

1. Consider a daily supplement of **1 - 5mg of folic acid** in severe cases of increased homocysteine.

   - A daily dose of **400mcg of Folic acid** as a maintenance dose can reduce homocysteine.

2. Consider a daily supplement of **50mg to 100mg of vitamin B6** (depending on severity)

3. Consider a daily supplement of **1-2.5mg of sub-lingual vitamin B12**.

4. Consider a daily supplement of **2g of Betaine HCl** may be beneficial in reducing homocysteine.

5. Increase the amount of **cereals and green leafy vegetables** you eat

For Those That Want To Treat Alzheimer's Disease and Dementia By Improving Their Brain Chemistry.

1. Reduce your levels of stress (if possible).

Stress increases the level of the hormone cortisol which damages the part of the brain involved with memory production. If feasible **consider taking up relaxation techniques such as relaxation CDs, hypnotherapy, tai-chi or yoga**.

2. Regulate the amount of alcohol that you drink.

One to three alcoholic drinks a day was associated with a 42% risk reduction of all types dementia by stimulating the release of the chemical acetylcholine in the hippocampus area of the brain – the area of the brain involved with converting short memories into long term memories – enhancing memory and learning.

3. Cut artificial sweeteners out of your diet.

- Aspartame stimulates the neurons of the brain to death, causing brain damage of varying degrees.

4. A daily dose of between **1.5 – 2.5mg of vitamin B12** sublingually may prove beneficial in reversing nerve damage associated with Alzheimer's disease and dementia and also regulate the action of the neurotransmitters in the brain.

5. A daily dose of up to **300mg vitamin B6** may prove beneficial in the treatment of most neurological conditions.

6. A daily dose of **15-20mg of Niacin** may prove beneficial in Alzheimer's disease and other dementias.

7. A daily dose of **12mg of Inositol** divided into 6 equal doses may be of benefit as Inositol plays an important role in brain cell communication and function, the regulation of brain chemicals (the neurotransmitters serotonin and acetylcholine are both regulated by inositol).

8. For regulation of acetylcholine the following may be beneficial:

- A daily supplementation of **800-100mg of Choline.**
- A supplement of up to **20 drops of Sage tincture** three times a day.
- A supplement of up to **1000mg of Lemon Balm a day** can be beneficial.
- A daily supplement of **800mg of Rosemary leaf** may be beneficial.

9. For general regulation of neurotransmitters the following may be beneficial:

- A **Ginkgo Biloba supplement of up to 200mg** a day.
- A daily supplement of **400mg of Ginseng extract**.

10. A **Galantamine supplement of 16 mg a day** can be beneficial in helping to regulate the brains neurotransmitters, prevent acetylcholine breakdown and prevent nerve cell death.

11. A **Magnesium supplement of 250-500mg a day** can be beneficial in improving the functioning of the brain and formation of nerve pathways.

12. A **Lithium Orotate (or Aspartate)** supplement may be beneficial in protecting the brain and preventing the normal brain shrinkage associated with age.

For Those That Want To Treat Alzheimer's Disease and Dementia
By Reducing the build Up Of Plaques.

1. A **Curcumin supplement of up to 1000mg a day** can be beneficial in suppressing oxidative damage, inflammation, cognitive deficits and amyloid accumulation by breaking up and untangling amyloid plaques. Curcumin may aggravate certain stomach and bile duct conditions and caution is advised if taking anticoagulant or anti-inflammatory drugs

2. A daily supplement of **800mg of Rosemary leaf** may be beneficial in slowing and reversing the build up of amyloid plaques.

3. **100mg of Myricetin** daily may be beneficial in reducing the build up amyloid plaques in Alzheimer's disease.

4. A dose of **250 mg of Ferulic Acid** may be beneficial in reducing the build up amyloid plaques.

5. **One to two 50mcg capsules of Huperzine A** may slow the build up amyloid plaques.
- Huperzine A has actions similar to other medications prescribed for Alzheimer's disease therefore you should consult your general practitioner before taking it.
- Any one suffering from high blood pressure should note take Huperzine A.

For Those That Want To Treat Alzheimer's Disease and Dementia By Taking Vitamin Supplements.

1. A daily dose of **2500-3000mg of vitamin C** may prove beneficial in reducing and slowing the effects of Alzheimer's and other dementias.

2. A daily dose of **800mg of vitamin E** may prove beneficial in reducing and slowing the effects of Alzheimer's and other dementias.

The above two vitamins have even greater effect if taken in conjunction.

3. A daily dose of **400mcg of Folic acid** as a maintenance dose and increasing this dose to 2,000mcg if you are showing signs of early dementia or have a family history of dementia.

4. A daily dose of between **1.5 – 2.5mg of vitamin B12** sublingually may prove beneficial in the treatment of Alzheimer's disease and other dementias.

5. A daily dose of up to **300mg vitamin B6** may prove beneficial in the treatment of most neurological conditions.

6. A daily dose of **15-20mg of Niacin** may prove beneficial in Alzheimer's disease and other dementias.

7. A daily dose of **12mg of Inositol** divided into 6 equal doses may be of benefit as Inositol plays an important role in brain cell communication and function, the regulation of brain chemicals (the neurotransmitters serotonin and acetylcholine are both regulated by inositol).

8. A daily supplementation of **800-100mg of Choline** should provide beneficial results in correcting the brains levels of acetylcholine.

For Those That Want To Treat Alzheimer's Disease and Dementia
By Taking Herbal Supplements.

1. A **Curcumin supplement of up to 1000mg a day** can be beneficial in suppressing oxidative damage, inflammation, cognitive deficits and amyloid accumulation by breaking up and untangling amyloid plaques. Curcumin may aggravate certain stomach and bile duct conditions and caution is advised if taking anticoagulant or anti-inflammatory drugs

2. A **Ginkgo Biloba supplement of up to 200mg** a day can be beneficial.

3. A daily supplement of **400mg of Ginseng extract** can be beneficial for those suffering from Alzheimer's disease and other dementias.

The above two herbs have even greater effect if taken in conjunction.

4. A supplement of up to **20 drops of Sage tincture** three times a day can be beneficial.

5. A **Lemon Balm supplement of up to 1000mg a day** can be beneficial.

6. A **Galantamine supplement of 16 mg a day** can be beneficial. A suggested dose is 8mg in the morning and 8mg at night.
7. **100mg of Myricetin** daily may be beneficial.

8. **10mg of Vinpocetine** three times a day may be beneficial for those suffering from vascular dementia or Alzheimer's disease.

9. A dose of **250 mg of Ferulic Acid** may be beneficial in the treatment of Alzheimer's disease and other neurodegenerative disorders.

10. **One to two 50mcg capsules of Huperzine A** daily will improve memory and may slow the progression of Alzheimer's disease and other dementias.

- Huperzine A has actions similar to other medications prescribed for Alzheimer's disease therefore you should consult your general practitioner before taking it.
- Any one suffering from high blood pressure should note take Huperzine A.

11. **400-500mg of Bacopa extract** daily should prove beneficial for all cognitive disorders.

For Those That Want To Treat Alzheimer's Disease and Dementia
By Taking Mineral and / or Other Supplements.

1. A **Malic Acid supplement of 1000mg a day** can be beneficial.

2. A **Magnesium supplement of 250-500mg a day** can be beneficial.

3. A **supplement of 200-400mcg of Selenium** a day can be beneficial.

4. A supplement of no greater than **5mg of Boron** may be of benefit in improving memory and cognition.

5. A **Lithium Orotate (or Aspartate)** supplement may be beneficial in protecting the brain and preventing damage associated with ageing.

Section
Seven

Resources

I hope that the material that you have now read has given you not only an insight but also hope in the knowledge that there are plenty of things that can be done to help improve and slow the affects and progression of Alzheimer's disease.

Sometimes however knowledge on its own is not enough.

The following pages contain a list of many support organisations, associations, books and websites that will also be able to offer you help and support and reassure you that you are not facing any difficulties, uncertainties and troubles alone.

These sites (although not listed in any order) will between them be able to provide you with any further information and help that you may need.

Alzheimer's Disease International

Alzheimer's Disease International is the umbrella organisation of Alzheimer's associations around the world offering support and information to people with dementia and their carers. It's aim is to help establish and strengthen Alzheimer's associations throughout the world and raise global awareness about Alzheimer's disease and all other causes of dementia.

Alzheimer's Disease International
64 Great Suffolk Street
London
SE1 0BL
UK
Tel: +44 20 79810880
Fax: +44 20 79282357
Email: info@alz.co.uk

Alzheimer's Society.

The Alzheimer's Society is a membership organisation, which works to improve the quality of life of people affected by dementia in England, Wales and Northern Ireland. Many of their 25,000 members have personal experience of dementia, as carers, health professionals or people with dementia themselves. The site offers information and advice to people with Alzheimer's disease and their carers. Information sheets, books and videos on all aspects of caring for someone with dementia are available.

Gordon House
10 Greencoat Place
London
SW1 1PH

Tel: 08453000336
Email info@Alzheimers.org.uk
Website www.Alzheimers.org.uk

Alzheimer Scotland - Action on Dementia.

Alzheimer Scotland helps people with dementia, their carers and families. Their members include carers, relatives, people with dementia, professionals, groups and organisations. Their aims are to improve public policies for people with dementia and their carers in Scotland and to provide and secure the provision of high-quality services both for people with dementia and for their carers.

22 Drumsheugh Gardens
Edinburgh
Scotland
EH3 &RN

Tel helpline: 0800 808 3000
Fax: 0131 243 1450
Email: Alzheimer@alzscot.org
Website: http://www.alzscot.org/pages/sitemap.htm

Western Alzheimer's Foundation

The Western Alzheimers Foundation promotes awareness of Alzheimer's disease and its impact on families through education, talks, promotional material and support group meetings.

Mount Street
Claremorris
Co. Mayo
Ireland

Tel: +353 94 62480
Fax: +353 94 62560
Email: westalz@iol.ie
Website: http://www.westernalzheimer.ie/

Age Concern

Their mission is to promote the well-being of all older people and to help make later life a fulfilling and enjoyable experience by supporting all people over 50 in the UK, ensuring that they get the most from life. They provide essential services such as day care and information. They also campaign on issues like age discrimination and pensions, and work to influence public opinion and government policy about older people.

Age Concern England

1268 London Road
London
SW16 4ER
Tel: 020 87657200
Email: acw@ace.org.uk
Website: www.ageconcern.org.uk

Age Concern Cymru (Wales)

4th Floor
1 Catherdral Road
Cardiff
Wales
CF11 9SD

Tel: 02920371566
Email: inquiries@accymru.org.uk
Website: www.accymru.org.uk

Age Concern Northern Ireland.

3Lower Crescent
Belfast
Northern Ireland
BT7 1NR

Tel: 02890 245729
Advice line: 02890 325055 (weekdays 9.30am-1pm)
Email: info@ageconcernnni.org

Benefits Enquiry Line (BEL)

The Benefit Enquiry Line is a benefits help line for people with disabilities, carers and representatives. They offer confidential advice and information on benefits and how to claim them. In addition to giving advice they are also able to send out an extensive range of leaflets and claim packs to customers. As a national service they serve the whole of England, Scotland and Wales.

Benefit Enquiry Line
Victoria House
9th Floor
Ormskirk Road
Preston
Lancashire
PR1 2QP

Tel: 0800 88 22 00
Fax: 01772 23 89 53
Email: Bel-Customer-Services@dwp.gsi.gov.uk

Candid (Counselling and Diagnosis in Dementia).

CANDID is a unique service, established at the National Hospital for Neurology and Neurosurgery. It arose out of experience gained from a specialist young onset dementia clinic. Its aims are to increase accessibility to advice, diagnosis and counselling for patients, their families and involved health professionals. The service is aimed particularly, but not exclusively, at patients with young onset dementia.

CANDID operates a general advice and information service, accessed by telephone and electronic mail, providing information for professionals, carers and families.

The National Hospital for Neurology and Neurosurgery
Queens Square
London
WC1N 3BG

Tel: 020 7829 8773
Fax: 0870 132 0447
Email: enquires@dementia.icon.ucl.ac.uk
Website: dementia.ion.ucl.ac.uk
Information and dementia resource centre:
http://dementia.ion.ucl.ac.uk/DRG_Website/Candid/Candi
d_factsheets/facts2.htm

Carers UK

Carers UK is the voice of carers, it is a support organisation for carers whose aims are to make people recognise the true value of carers' contribution to society and get carers the practical, financial and emotional support they need.

Carers UK
32-36 Loman Street
Southwark
London SE1 0EE
Tel: 020 7922 8000
Email: info@carersuk.org
Website: www.carersuk.org

Carers Scotland
91 Mitchell Street
Glasgow G1 3LN
Tel: 0141 221 9141
Email: info@carerscotland.org
Website: www.carerscotland.org

Carers Wales
River House
Ynsbridge Court
Gwaelod-y-Garth
Cardiff CF15 9SS
Tel: 029 2081 1370
Email: info@carerswales.org
Website: www.carerswales.org

Carers Northern Ireland
58 Howard Street
Belfast BT1 6PJ

Tel: 028 9043 9843
Email: info@carersni.org
Website: www.carersni.org

Crossroads - Caring for Carers.

The aim of the Crossroads service is to give time –
to improve the lives of carers by giving them time to be
themselves and have a break from their caring
responsibilities. Their aim is to provide a reliable service,
tailored to meet the individual needs of each carer and the
person they are caring for. They have schemes in most
parts of England and Wales, which provide a range of
services to meet local needs.

10 Regent Place
Rugby
Warwickshire
CV21 2PN

Tel: 01788 573653
Website: www.crossroads.org.uk

DIAL UK
(Disablement Information and Advice Line).

DIAL UK is a national organisation for a network of approximately 130 local Disability Information and Advice Line services (DIALs) run by and for disabled people. Their information and advice services are based throughout the UK and provide information and advice to disabled people and others on all aspects of living with a disability.

St Catherine's
Tickhill Road
Doncaster
DN4 8QN

Tel: 01302 310123
Fax: 01302310404
Email: enquirires@dialuk.org.uk

Help The Aged.

Help The Aged mission is to work for disadvantaged older people in the UK and around the world. We research their needs, campaign for their social and political rights, and provide services which alleviate hardship today and prevent deprivation tomorrow.

207-221 Pentonville Road
London
N1 9UZ
Tel: 020 7278 1114
Email: info@helptheaged.org.uk
Website: www.helptheaged.org.uk

MIND.

Mind is the leading mental health charity in England and Wales. They work to create a better life for everyone with experience of mental distress by:

- advancing the views, needs and ambitions of people with mental health problems
- challenging discrimination and promoting inclusion
- influencing policy through campaigning and education
- inspiring the development of quality services which reflect expressed need and diversity
- achieving equal rights through campaigning and education.

Broadway 15-19
London
E15 4BQ

Tel: 020 8519 2122, F: 020 8522 1725
Email: contact@mind.org.uk
Website: www.mind.org.uk

The Princess Royal Trust for Carers

The Princess Royal Trust for Carers is the largest provider of comprehensive carers support services in the UK. Through its unique network of 133 independently managed Carers' Centres , 83 young carers services and interactive websites, Carers.org and YC Net, The Trust currently provides quality information, advice and support services to almost 310,000 carers, including over 15,500 young carers.

In addition, The Trust also acts independently in the interests of carers through:

- Research, development and consultation
- Influence on national, regional and local policy
- Partnerships with other national organisations
- Information through our interactive websites, providing advice and access to support groups

London Office
The Princess Royal Trust for Carers
Unit 14, Bourne Court
Southend Road
Woodford Green
Essex
IG8 8HD

Tel: 0844 800 4361
Fax: 0844 800 4362
Email: info@carers.org

Glasgow Office
The Princess Royal Trust for Carers
Charles Oakley House
125 West Regent Street
Glasgow
G2 2SD

Tel: (0141) 221 5066
Fax: (0141) 221 4623
Email: Info Scotland (infoscotland@carers.org)

Northern Office
Suite 6, Oak House,
High Street,
Chorley PR7 1DW

Tel: (01257) 234 070
Fax: (01257) 234 105
Email: Info Chorley (infochorley@carers.org)

Wales Office
Victoria House
250 Cowbridge Road East
Canton
Cardiff
CF5 1GZ

Tel: 02920 221788
Email: Info Wales (infowales@carers.org)

RADAR
(The Royal Association for Disability And Rehabilitation)

RADAR is a national network of disability organisations and disabled people. They represent their members by fast-tracking your opinions and concerns to policy-makers and legislators in Westminster and Whitehall, and launching their own campaigns to promote equality for all disabled people. Formed in 1977 as the Royal Association for Disability and Rehabilitation, RADAR is a national organisation run by and working for disabled people. They have a membership of over 800 disability organisations and individuals.

12 City Forum
250 City Road
London
EC1V 8AF

Tel: 020 7250 3222
Minicom: 020 7250 4119
Email: radar@radar.org.uk
Website: www.radar.org.uk

The Relatives & Residents Association

The Relatives & Residents Association exists to provide a consumer voice to promote the well-being and represent the interests of older people in residential care settings. They offer advice, support and information to help potential residents, their families and friends to be better informed regarding many aspects of care including:

- Rights
- Entitlements
- National Minimum Standards
- Finding a care home
- Local Authority and NHS obligations towards residents
- Advice on how to deal with care concerns or abuse

They offer an advice line (via phone, email or post) which is open to anyone and offers whatever support is necessary.

24 The Ivories
6-18 Northampton Street
London N1 2HY
Website http://www.relres.org/index.php

Email: info@relres.org
Tel: 020 7359 8148
Fax: 020 7226 6603
Advice Line: 020 7359 8136 (Monday - Friday 9:30 - 4:30pm)

Books

Elder Rage or Take my Father... Please: How To Survive Caring For Ageing Parents by Jacqueline Marcell.

This is a true story, written with compassion, heart and humour that will help you realise that you're not alone with your countless frustrations and conflicting emotions when coping with an elderly loved one who is experiencing memory loss and mood swings. This incredible roller coaster ride is a can't-put-it-down page-turner, as well as a how-to guide for struggling caregivers. Triumph with this devoted daughter as she mends her frail mother and finally turns her rebellious "Jekyll & Hyde" father around, with the right doctors and medications, adult day care, and creative behaviour modification - at 85 years old!

New Hope for People with Alzheimer's and their Caregivers: Traditional and Complementary Solutions by Porter Shimer.

All those impacted by Alzheimer's disease can improve their quality of life, starting today. This helpful book dispels the myths and clearly lays out the truth about Alzheimer's and offers practical solutions for not only those who have the disease, but also their families and their caregivers. Amongst other things it includes information on:

- The signs, symptoms, and proper diagnosis of Alzheimer's.
- Living with Alzheimer's and providing the best possible care.
- Cutting-edge research, including advances in biotechnology and genetics.
- The latest conventional drugs and effective natural treatments.

Alzheimer's Early Stages:
First Steps for Family, Friends and Caregivers
by Daniel Kuhn.

This book helps families in developing a philosophy of care, offering clear, current information on the nature of the illness along with anecdotes drawn from the author's own practice and first-person caregiver accounts. Throughout the book the author stresses the importance of sharing the care by involving others. Especially valuable is the extensive resource list of web sites, organizations, and references to consumer and professional literature.

Learning to Speak Alzheimer's: The New Approach to Living Positively with Alzheimer's Disease
by Joanne Koenig-Coste

Few conditions upon first diagnosis strike such terror into victims and relatives as Alzheimer's disease. The dementia that is its best-known symptom can provoke feelings of helplessness and despair, coupled with fear that the patient will inevitably suffer loss of dignity and self-respect. For over 30 years, the author has practised a communication-based form of care. She shows how, by following a few straightforward and simple ideas, the quality of life for Alzheimer's sufferers can be dramatically improved, and their dignity and self-respect renewed.

Rehabilitation capitalizes on the remaining emotions and skills of the patient and offers chances to feel successful by reaching past the recognized losses, ignoring the failures and rejoicing in whatever still defines the essential humanity of the sufferer.

Perhaps as importantly, it also suggests ways that the carers can care for themselves. This text provides a practical guide to coping with a cruel disease. It offers information, understanding and advice, but above all it offers a message of hope based on respect, common sense and quiet dignity.

The Memory Cure:
The Safe, Scientifically Proven Breakthrough That
Can Slow, Halt, or Even Reverse Age-Related Memory
Loss by Thomas Crook Ph.D and Brenda Adderly

If you're suffering from the effects of age-associated memory impairment (AAMI), you're in a crowd of millions. But according to The Memory Cure, phosphatidylserine (PS), a soy-based nutritional supplement, has been scientifically proven to help people recapture their slipping memories.

The Memory Cure tells you everything you ever wanted to know about memory, making scientific information lucid and accessible. Memory expert Thomas Crook and health researcher-writer Brenda Adderly discuss the different types of memory, why we forget, and how PS works to invigorate memory. The authors also present a variety of memory-enhancing tips, techniques, and games. They discuss lifestyle choices that can affect memory, such as foods, supplements, exercise, and stress management.

Websites

www.alz.org

The Alzheimer's Association is an American site that is one of the largest voluntary health organizations dealing with Alzheimer's care, support and research. Their vision is a world without Alzheimer's disease and their aims are to eliminate the condition through research, whilst providing and enhancing the care and support of all affected.

For those not resident in the USA they provide access to an on-line community for people to share their experiences of Alzheimer's disease and find support and friendship with others affected by the illness. Their home page also offers some useful on-line information about the condition as well as information for carers.

www.alzheimer-europe.org

Alzheimer Europe is a non-profit organisation which aims to improve the care and treatment of Alzheimer's patients through collaborations between its member associations in order to become the main information centre for all organisations working in the field of Alzheimer's. By doing this Alzheimer Europe hopes to answer a growing need (especially among the community of people affected by the existence of the disease) by exchanging experiences, knowledge as well as collaborating on new approaches so that the best information regarding all aspects of the condition is available throughout Europe and beyond.

Their website (accessed though the links on the left hand side of the home page) contains a vast array of information regarding Alzheimer's disease from both the aspect of the sufferer and carer as well as information on legal issues, benefits and the help that is available.

www.dementia.com

This site is again aimed at the European advances in the medical advances and treatment of Alzheimer's disease. In fact there is a lot of medical and research information to be accessed from this site as it is published by Janssen-Pharmaceutica NV.

However this site does not approach the condition from a purely medical aspect and it does also have some very good information as it brings you the latest news on developments in care-giving (with good information for those with family or friends that are affected by the condition) that is of value to carers.

www.healingwell.com/alzheimers

This is another excellent all round site providing information on many health related conditions and not just Alzheimer's disease. The Alzheimer's section in particular offers useful articles, book extracts and an excellent on-line community with over 50,000 members as well as a very in depth resources page for further information regarding alternative treatments and approaches.

Section Eight

References

Section 2

1. "Apolipoprotein E4 Allele, Elevated Mid-life Cholesterol and Systolic Blood Pressure are Independent Risk Factors for Late-Life Alzheimer's Disease" Abstract from the International Conference on Alzheimer's Disease and Related Disorders (ICADRD) 2002.

2. "Diabetes Mellitus and Risk of Alzheimer Disease and Decline in Cognitive Function." Zoe Arvanitakis, MD et al. Archives of Neurology 2004;61:661-666.

3. "Amyloid beta oligomers induce impairment of neuronal insulin receptors." William L. Klein et al. Journal of the Federation of American Societies for Experimental Biology. 2008 22: 246-260; published online as doi:10.1096/fj.06-7703com

4. "Effect of a clinical stroke on the risk of dementia in a prospective cohort." Gamaldo A et al. Neurology 2006 Oct 24; 67:1363-9.

5. "Relationship of vascular risk to the progression of Alzheimer disease." Regan C et al. Neurology 2006 Oct 24; 67:1357-62.

6. "15-year longitudinal study of blood pressure and dementia." Skoog, I et al. Lancet. 1996 Apr 27;347(9009):1141-5

7. "Midlife blood pressure and dementia: the Honolulu-Asia ageing study." Launer, L.J. et al. Neurobiology of Ageing. 2000 Jan-Feb;21(1):49-55.

8. "Antihypertensive Medication Use and Incident Alzheimer Disease." Ara, S. et al. Archives of Neurology 2006, 63 (DOI: 10.1001/archneur.63.5.noc60013

9. "High Cholesterol in Your 40s Increases Risk of Alzheimer's Disease." Alina Solomon, M.D. American Academy of Neurology 60th Anniversary Annual Meeting in Chicago, April 12–19, 2008

10. "Elevated levels of cholesterol play an even greater role in development of Alzheimer's, study shows" Press release, Georgetown University Medical Centre

11. "Function of b-Amyloid in Cholesterol Homeostasis: A Lead to Neurotoxicity" Abstract P3-313, 2002 Annual Meeting of The Endocrine Society

12. "Decreased prevalence of Alzheimer's disease associated with 3-hydroxy-3-methylglutaryl coenzyme A reductase inhibitors." Wolozin B, Kellman W, Rousseau P, et al. Archives of Neurology. 2000;57:1439-1443.

13. "Statins and the risk of dementia." Jick H, Zomberg G.L., Jick S.S., et al. Lancet. 2000;356:1627-1631

14. "Statin use and the risk of incident dementia: the Cardiovascular Health Study." Rea T.D., Breitner J.C. et al Archives of Neurology. 2005 Jul;62(7):1047-51.

15. "Reversing atherosclerosis: An interview with Dr. Anthony Verlangieri." Passwater, Richard A. Whole Foods 15(8):27-30 (Aug. 1992)

16. "Vitamin E and Carotenoids Protect Arteries from Cholesterol Deposits." Interview With Dr. Hermann Esterbauer By Richard A. Passwater Ph.D

17. "Reduced Risk of Alzheimer Disease in Users of Antioxidant Vitamin Supplements: The Cache County Study." Zandi, P.P., et al. Archives of Neurology. 2004;61:82-88.

18. "Plasma Homocysteine as a Risk Factor for Dementia and Alzheimer's Disease." Seshadri, S. et al New England Journal of Medicine. Vol. 346:476-483. No.7 2002.

19. "Vascular factors predict rate of progression in Alzheimer disease." Mielke, M.M., et al. Neurology 2007 69: 1850-1858.

20. "Atherosclerosis, apolipoprotein E, and prevalence of dementia and Alzheimer's disease in the Rotterdam Study." Hofman, A. et al. Lancet. 1997 Apr 19;349(9059):1174.

21. "Circle of Willis Atherosclerosis Is a Risk Factor for Sporadic Alzheimer's Disease" Roher, A.E., et al. Arteriosclerosis, Thrombosis, and Vascular Biology. 2003;23:2055

22. "Larger Belly in Mid-Life Increases Risk of Dementia" American Academy of Neurology, Press Release, 3/26/08, eurekalert.org

23. "Exercise Is Associated with Reduced Risk for Incident Dementia among Persons 65 Years of Age and Older" Larson, E.B., et al. Annals of Internal Medicine, Jan. 2006,Vol: 144, No.2 Pages 73-81.

24. "Exercise and activity level in Alzheimer's disease: a potential treatment focus." McCurry, T.L., et al. Journal of Rehabilitation Research & Development 1998; 35: Pgs 411-9.

25. "Prevalence of Alzheimer's disease and vascular dementia: Association with education. The Rotterdam study." Ott, A. et al. British Medical Journal. 1995;310:970–973.

26. "Education and the incidence of dementia in a large population-based study: The Rotterdam Study." Ott ,A. et al. Neurology. 1999;52:663–666.

27. "Influence of leisure activity on the incidence of Alzheimer's disease." Scarmeas, N. et al. Neurology. 2001;57:2236–2242.

28. "Cognitive activity and incident AD in a population-based sample of older persons." Wilson, R.S. Et al. Neurology. 2002;59:1910–1914.

29. "Use it or lose it: Engaged lifestyle as a buffer of cognitive decline in ageing?" Hultsch, D.F.,et al. Psychology and Aging. 1999;14:245–263.

30. "Glucocorticoids Increase Amyloid-β and Tau Pathology in a Mouse Model of Alzheimer's Disease." Green, K.N., et al. The Journal of Neuroscience, August 30, 2006, 26(35):9047-9056.

31. "Smoking and risk of dementia and Alzheimer's disease in a population-based cohort study: the Rotterdam Study." Ott, A. et al. Lancet 1998. Vol. 351, no. 9119, pgs. 1840-1843.

32. "Alcohol and tobacco consumption as risk factors for Alzheimer's disease: a collaborative re-analysis of case-control studies." Graves, A.B., et al. EURODEM Risk Factors Research Group. International Journal of Epidemiology, Vol. 20, S48-S57

33. "Alcohol consumption and risk of dementia: the Rotterdam Study." Breteler, M. et al. The Lancet, Volume 359, Issue 9303, Pages 281 - 286 .

Section 3

1. "Caloric Intake and the Risk of Alzheimer's Disease." Luchsinger, J.A., et al. Archives of Neurology 2002;59:1258-1263

2. "Limited Alzheimer-Type Neurodegeneration in Experimental Obesity and Type 2 Diabetes Mellitus." Moroz, N., et al. Journal of Alzheimer's Disease. 2008. 15(1), 29-44.

3. "A ketogenic diet reduces amyloid beta 40 and 42 in a mouse model of Alzheimer's disease" Van der Auwera, A., et al. Nutrition & Metabolism.

4. "Sugary drinks linked to Alzheimer's, says study," www.foodnavigator.com, 12/10/07

5. "The suppression of age-related accumulation of lipid peroxides in rat brain by administration of rooibos tea (Aspalathus linearis)". Inanami, O. et al., (1995) Neuroscience Letters, 196, (1-2): 85-8.

6. "Coffee consumption is inversely associated with cognitive decline in elderly European men: the FINE Study" van Gelder, B.M. et al. European Journal of Clinical Nutrition, August 2007.

7. "Does caffeine intake protect from Alzheimer's disease?." Maia, L., de Mendonca, A. European Journal of Neurology. 9(4):377-382, July 2002.

8. "Fruit and Vegetable Juices and Alzheimer's Disease: The Kame Project." Dai, Q., et al. The American Journal of Medicine. 2008. Volume 119, Issue 9, Pages 751 – 759.

9. "The Impact of the Use of Statins on the Prevalence of Dementia and the Progression of Cognitive Impairment" Hajjara, I., et al. The Journals of Gerontology Series A: Biological Sciences and Medical Sciences 2002. 57:M414-M418

10. Statins and the risk of dementia . Jick, H., et al. The Lancet, Volume 356 , Issue 9242 , Pages 1627 – 1631

11. "Effects of lovastatin on cognitive function and psychological well-being." Muldoon, M. F., et al. American Journal of Medicine. 108:538–546, 2000.

12. "Randomized trial of the effects of simvastatin on cognitive functioning in hypercholesterolemic adults." Muldoon, M. F., et al. American Journal of Medicine. 117:823–829, 2004.

13. "Low HDL Cholesterol Is a Risk Factor for Deficit and Decline in Memory in Midlife: The Whitehall II Study." Singh-Manoux, A., et al. Arteriosclerosis, Thrombosis, and Vascular Biology. 2008;28: Pages1556-62

14. "Headache and CNS white matter abnormalities associated with gluten sensitivity." Hadjivassiliou, M., et al. Neurology. 2001 Feb 13;56(3):385-8.

15. "Dietary Docosahexaenoic Acid and Docosapentaenoic Acid Ameliorate Amyloid-ß and Tau Pathology via a Mechanism Involving Presenilin 1 Levels" The Journal of Neuroscience, Vol. 27, No. 16, 4/18/07.

16. "Mental Illness – The Nutrition Connection. Carl Pfeiffer and Patrick Holford." ION Press, London. 1996

Section 4

1. "Low plasma vitamin C in Alzheimer patients despite an adequate diet." Riviere, S. et al., International Journal of Geriatric Psychiatry 1998, vol.13, n°11, pages 749-754 (27 ref.)

2. "Relation of the tocopherol forms to incident Alzheimer disease and to cognitive change." Morris, M.C., et al. American Journal of Clinical Nutrition, 2005. Vol. 81, No. 2, 508-514.

3. LA Times-Washington Post News Service. Lubbock Avalanche-Journal. 03/09/97 (http://www.lubbockonline.com/news/031097/ibuprofe.htm)

4. "Cognitive Function Over Time in the Alzheimer's Disease Anti-Inflammatory Prevention Trial (ADAPT)." Archives of Neurology, Early release article, 5/12/08, archneur.ama-assn.org

5. "Plasma Homocysteine as a Risk Factor for Dementia and Alzheimer's Disease." Seshadri, S., et al. The New England Journal of Medicine 2002; 346:2007-2008.

6. Natural Health Consultants: Methylcobalamin

7. "Vitamin B6 in clinical neurology." Bernstein, A.L. Annals of the New York Academy of Sciences 1990;585:250-60.

8. "Vitamin B6 status, deficiency and its consequences--an overview." Spinneker, A. et al. Nutrición Hospitalaria. 2007 Jan-Feb;22(1):7-24

9. "Dietary niacin and the risk of incident Alzheimer's disease and of cognitive decline." Morris, M.C., et al. Journal of Neurology Neurosurgery and Psychiatry 2004;75:1093-1099

10. "Inositol treatment of Alzheimer's disease: a doubleblind, cross-over placebo controlled trial." Barak, Y., et al. Progress in Neuro-Psychopharmacology & Biological Psychiatry. 20(4):729-35. 1996.

11. "Controlled trials of inositol in psychiatry." Levine, Journal of European Neuropsychopharmacology. 1997 May, 7:2, 147-55

12. "Methods and findings in experimental and clinical pharmacology." 1994, vol. 16, no. 8, pages 597-607.

13. "Association Between Serum Beta-Carotene Levels and Decline of Cognitive Function in High-Functioning Older Persons With or Without Apolipoprotein E 4 Alleles: MacArthur Studies of Successful Ageing." Hu, P., et al. The Journals of Gerontology Series A: Biological Sciences and Medical Sciences. Volume 61, Pages 616-620

14. "A randomized trial of beta carotene supplementation and cognitive function in men: the Physicians' Health Study II." Grodstein, F. et al., Archives of Internal Medicine. 2007 Nov 12;167(20):2167-8.

15. "Plasma carotenoid levels and cognitive performance in an elderly population: Results of an EVA study." Tasnime Akbaraly, N. et al., Journal of Gerontology: Medical Sciences 2007; 62A(3): 308-316

16. "Curcumin Inhibits Formation of Amyloid Oligomers and Fibrils and Binds Plaques and Reduces Amyloid in Vivo" Journal of Biological Chemistry, 2004 Dec 7. Yang F, et al., University of California Los Angeles, North Hills, CA

17. "Curcuminoids Enhance Amyloid-B by Macrophages of Alzheimer's Disease Patients" Journal of Alzheimer's Disease, Vol. 10, No. 1, September 2006.

18. "Curcumin Linked to Better Performance for Elderly Brains" Stephen Daniells, FoodNavigator, 10/27/06, foodnavigator.com

19. "Ginkgo Biloba for Cognitive Impairment and Dementia" Cochrane Review, Published in: The Cochrane Database of Systematic Reviews 2002, Issue 4.

20. "Ginkgo Improves Memory of Dementia Patients" Dr. Joseph Mercola, 11/2/02

21. "Reciprocal activity of ginsenosides in the production of proinflammatory repertoire, and their potential roles in neuroprotection in vivo." Joo, S.S., et al
Planta Medica 2005; 71(5): 476-481.

22. "Effect of ginseng saponins on beta-amyloid-suppressed acetylcholine release from rat hippocampal slices." Lee, T. F., et al. Planta Medica.

23. "Panax Ginseng Enhances Cognitive Performance in Alzheimer Disease." Lee, S. T., et al. Alzheimer's Disease and Associated Disorders

24. "Melissa officinalis extract in the treatment of patients with mild to moderate Alzheimer's disease: a double blind, randomised, placebo controlled trial." Akhondzadeh S, Noroozian M, et al. Journal of Clinical Pharmaceutical and Therapeutics 2003, 28(1): 53-59).

25. "Aromatherapy as a safe and effective treatment for the management of agitation in severe dementia: the results of a double-blind, placebo-controlled trial with Melissa." Ballard C.G, O'Brien J.T., Reichelt K, Perry E.K. Journal of Clinical Psychiatry. 2002;63(7):553-558.

26. "Melissa officinalis extract in the treatment of patients with mild to moderate Alzheimer's disease: a double blind, randomised, placebo controlled trial." Akhondzadeh S, Noroozian M, et al.Journal of Neurology, Neurosurgery and Psychiatry 2003, 74(7):863-866.

27. "Modulation of mood and cognitive performance following acute administration of Melissa officinalis (lemon balm)" Kennedy D.O., et al. Pharmacology Biochemistry and Behaviour 2002, 72(4): 953-964.

28. "The spice sage and its active ingredient rosmarinic acid protect PC12 cells from amyloid-{beta} peptide-induced neurotoxicity." Iuvone, T., et al. The Journal of Pharmacology and Experimental Therapeutics. 2006 Feb 22;

29. "Neurobehavioral and genotoxic aspects of rosmarinic acid." Pereira, P. et al. Pharmacological Research. 2005 Sept; 52(3):199-203.

30. www.fda.gov/cder/drug/infopage/galantamine/default.htm

31. "Galantamine for Alzheimer's disease and mild cognitive impairment." Loy C, Schneider L. *Cochrane Database of Systematic Reviews* 2001, Issue 1. Art. No.: CD001747. DOI: 10.1002/14651858.CD001747.pub3

32. "Galantamine prolonged-release formulation in the treatment of mild to moderate Alzheimer's disease." Brodaty H, Corey-Bloom J, Potocnik FC, et al. Dementia and Geriatric Cognitive Disorders. 2005; 20: 120-132.

33. "Peripheral and dual binding site inhibitors of acetylcholinesterase as neurodegenerative disease modifying agents." Isabel Dorronsoro, Ana Castro and Ana Martinez. Journal of Neural Transmission - Supplementum. 2002;(62): Pages 203-216.

34. "Nerve growth factor and galantamine ameliorate early signs of neurodegeneration in anti-nerve growth factor mice." Simona Capsoni, Sabina Giannotta, and Antonino Cattaneo. Proceedings of the National Academy of Sciences of the United States. 2002 September 17; 99(19): Pages 12432–12437.

35. "Potent anti-amyloidogenic and fibril-destabilizing effects of polyphenols in vitro: implications for the prevention and therapeutics of Alzheimer's disease." Ono, K., et al. Journal of Neurochemistry. 2003 Oct;87(1):Pages 172-81.

36. "Multifunction of myricetin on A beta: neuroprotection via a conformational change of A beta and reduction of A beta via the interference of secretases." Shimmyo, Y., et al. Journal of Neuroscience Research. 2008 Feb 1;86(2):368-77

37. "Pharmacology of nootropics and metabolically active compounds in relation to their use in dementia." Nicholson CD. Psychopharmacology (Berl) 1990;101(2):147-59

38. "In vivo protection of synaptosomes by ferulic acid ethyl ester (FAEE) from oxidative stress." Gururaj, G. et al. Neurochemistry International 2006 48: 318-27.

39. "In vivo protective effects of ferulic acid ethyl ester against amyloid-beta peptide 1-42-i." Perluigi, M., et al. Journal of Neuroscience Research (2006) 84: 418-26.

40. "Cholinesterase inhibiting withanolides from Withania somnifera." Choudhary, M.I., et al. Chemical and Pharmaceutical Bulletin (Tokyo). 2004 Nov;52(11):1358-61.

41. "Neuritic regeneration and synaptic reconstruction induced by withanolide A.£ Kuboyama, T., et al. British Journal of Pharmacology, 2005 Vol. 144, 961–971

42. "Huperzine A: Potential Therapeutic Agent for Alzheimer's Disease." Bai, D.L., Tang X.C. And He, X.C. Current Medicinal Chemistry 2000 Mar;7(3):355-74

43. "Comparative studies of huperzine A, E2020, and tacrine on behaviour and cholinesterase activities." Cheng, D.H. and Tang X.C. Pharmacology Biochemistry and Behaviour. 1998;60:377-386.

44. "CNS acetylcholine receptor activity in European medicinal plants traditionally used to improve failing memory". Wake, G. et al. Journal of Ethnopharmacology. 2000 Feb; 69(2): 105-14.

45. "Search for constituents with neurotrophic factor-potentiating activity from the medicinal plants of Paraguay and Thailand". Li, Y and Ohizumi, Y. Yakugaku Zasshi - Journal of the Pharmaceutical Society of Japan. 2004. vol. 124(7), pages 417-24

46. "Screening of traditionally used Lebanese herbs for neurological activities." Salah, S.M. And Jäger, A.K. Journal of Ethnopharmacology. 2005 Feb 10;97(1):145-9.

47. "Fosfatidilserina e disturbi della memoria nell-anziano" Nerozzi, D. La clinica Terapeutica. 1987. Vol.120. Pages 399-404.

48. "Phosphatidylserine in the treatment of Alzheimer's disease: Results of Multicentre Study." Amaducci, L. Psychopharmacology Bulletin. 1988. Vol. 24(1). Pages 130-134.

Section 5

1. Canadian Journal of Public Health 1992; 83: 97-100.

2. Neuroscience Research Communications, 1993, 13:2, 99-104, Society for Neuroscience Annual Meeting; San Diego, CA, 1995, Brain Research 1998; 784: 284-298

3. "The dangers posed by Teflon." Nature 2001; 412: 312- 324.

4. "Trace element imbalances in isolated subcellular fractions of Alzheimer's disease brains." By David Wenstrup, William D. Ehmann, and William R. Markesbery. Brain Research, No 533, 1990, pp. 125-130.

5. Federation of American Societies for Experimental Biology, 75th Annual Meeting, 21-25 April 1991

6. "Is there any relationship between aluminium and Alzheimer's disease?" Gunther L. Eichhorn. Experimental Gerontology Volume 28, Issues 4-5, July-October 1993, Pages 493-498

7. "Selenium Level and Cognitive Function in Rural Elderly Chinese." Gao, S., et al American Journal of Epidemiology 2007 165(8):955-965; doi:10.1093/aje/kwk073

8. "Treatment of Alzheimer's Disease By Zinc Compounds." Constantinidis, J. Drug Development Research 1992; 27: pgs. 1-14

9. "Dietary supplementation with zinc sulphate, sodium selenite and fatty acids in early dementia of Alzheimer's type." van Rhijn, A.G., Prior, C.A., Corrigan, F.M. Journal of Nutritional Medicine. Vol. 1, no. 4, pp. 259-266. 1990.

10. "Trace element imbalances in isolated subcellular fractions of Alzheimer's disease brains." By David Wenstrup, William D. Ehmann, and William R. Markesbery. Brain Research, No 533, 1990, pp. 125-130.

11. "Dietary Copper and High Saturated and trans Fat Intakes Associated With Cognitive Decline." Morris et al, Archives of Neurology.2006;63:1085-1088.

12. "Cognitive decline correlates with low plasma concentrations of copper in patients with mild to moderate Alzheimer's disease." Journal of Alzheimer's disease, Vol. 8, Issue 1. 2005

13. "In Vivo Evaluation of Brain Iron in Alzheimer Disease Using Magnetic Resonance Imaging" Bartzokis, G., et al. Archives of General Psychiatry. 2000;57:47-53.

14. "Heme deficiency may be a factor in the mitochondrial and neuronal decay of ageing." Atamna, H., et al. Proceedings of the National Academy of Sciences November 12, 2002, vol. 99, no. 23, 14807-14812

15. "Lithium-induced increase in human brain grey matter." Moore et al. The Lancet, Volume 356, Issue 9237, Pages 1241-1242

16. "Lithium inhibits Alzheimer's disease-like tau protein phosphorylation in neurons." Muñoz-Montaño et al, Federation of European Biochemical Societies Letters, 1997 – Elsevier Pages 1-6.

17. "Pathways to the decisive extension of the human specific lifespan". Bjorksten, J. Journal of the American Geriatrics Society, 1977 a, 25: 396-399.